霊
気

Degrees of Reiki

Maureen J. Kelly

LOTUS PRESS

P. O. BOX 325
TWIN LAKES, WI 53181
USA

DISCLAIMER
This book is not intended to treat, diagnose or prescribe. The information contained herein is in no way to be considered a substitute for your own good common sense, or as a substitute for a consultation with a duly licensed health care professional.

First Edition, 2002
Printed in the United States of America

LIBRARY OF CONGRESS CATALOGING-IN-PUBLICATION DATA
Kelly, Maureen J.
Degrees of Reiki
ISBN: 0-940985-56-X
1. Subject   I. Title
Library of Congress Control Number: 2002110948

Cover, page design and layout: Kerry P. Hopper, KPComm

Published By:
Lotus Press
P.O. Box 325
Twin Lakes, Wisconsin 53181 USA
Website: www.lotuspress.com
E-mail: lotuspress@lotuspress.com
(800) 824-6396

Table of Contents

From the Author:

I remember being intrigued and excited when an Aunt first told me about Reiki. I listened to her story and at the end I just had to know more about this magical energy that helped her overcome the pain and suffering of arthritis. The previous time I had visited with her she was using two walking sticks and trying her best not to let her misery show. Five years later, at the age of 80, she was happy and interested in everyone around her and walking without any assistance. My Aunt never became attuned to Reiki, but she had a Reiki treatment almost every week for the rest of her life. Her brother-in-law then told his story of how he cried when he walked because of arthritis in his feet and was expected to go into a wheelchair until he attended a 1st Degree Reiki class. As he treated himself each day with Reiki the pain diminished and he was able to lead a full and interesting life.

For me Reiki has been a wonder-filled journey, moving me into the unknown and returning me to the familiar of my life. At each obstacle, twist and turn I have been prompted to use Reiki to heal myself, keep moving forward, keep learning and keep discovering what life and Reiki are all about. When I trust the energy known as Reiki I find the process is easier and more fluid, often moving me on without my needing to know where I was going or why. I now cannot contemplate not having Reiki flowing through my hands and being available whenever I need it. I have been doing Reiki since 1992 and it remains intriguing and exciting.

This book looks at how I present Reiki to my students and the different Reiki classes that I teach. It is not the only way to teach Reiki, it is simply my way. If you choose to use this book I recommend you treat it as a guideline and take from it what you find to be interesting and helpful.

Although I have tried to make this book as comprehensive as possible it is not a "complete" book of Reiki. For it to be so would mean the energy was finite. Reiki will always continue to open up new experiences, possibilities and vistas. The longer we use Reiki the more we discover and the more there is to write about.

Thanks

I would especially like to acknowledge and thank Reiki Master Marie Angelo for the contribution she made to the editing and proof-reading of this book.

In 1993 my Mother attended a 1st Degree Reiki class where Tibetan Bells were played during attunements. She had received so much relief from Reiki treatments a friend and I had given her that she decided she would learn how to do Reiki as well. I would like to thank my Mother for sharing the poem she received immediately after her first Reiki attunement.

Prelude to Reiki

Vibrations from the bells

Urge me to explore

My Inner Depths of being

This, I've never done before

Warm and gentle hands

Help to guide me on my way

And pass to me the gift of healing

For ever and a day.

—PATRICIA KELLY

Chapter One

1st Degree Reiki

Hope your Reiki journey

Is a long and happy one

Full of adventure, discovery, healing

Full of pleasure and full of joy

ACKNOWLEDGEMENTS

My thanks go to my late Aunt, Mrs. Elizabeth Wakeling, for telling me about Reiki; to Reiki Master Gloria Warrender for giving me my first Reiki treatments; to Reiki Master Victoria Sinclair, for teaching me 1st Degree Reiki; to Reiki Master Lynne Walker for facilitating the Reiki Support Group I attended from 1992 to 1994; and to Reiki Master Tina Webb for giving me the 1st Degree Reiki attunements again that moved me on to 2nd Degree Reiki. And my thanks go to all my 1st Degree Reiki students who taught me so much through the questions they asked.

WHEN, WHERE AND HOW TO LEARN 1ST DEGREE REIKI

Reiki is taught by Reiki Masters in a series of steps, known as degrees. Attending a 1st Degree Reiki class is probably the biggest step you will take with Reiki. People often need to ask questions, read books and experience

Reiki Treatments before attending a Reiki Class. Once you have been attuned to Reiki you have the ability to channel the universal life force energy for the rest of your life. 1st Degree Reiki attunements cannot be reversed. Therefore it must be your decision to learn Reiki, not someone else's. You will know when you want to be attuned to Reiki because you will become excited about the idea or co-incidences and synchronicity will lead you to a Reiki class.

The Internet has many websites that advertise Reiki classes. These can be found by doing a search using the word Reiki. Many Reiki Masters leave pamphlets at their local Health Food shop, New Age bookstore or public library. Others advertise in magazines or newspapers. By far the most popular way of hearing about Reiki is from someone who has already attended a Reiki class. Once you know who to contact about a class phone, email or write to them and ask about their classes and if they teach near where you live. If they don't, ask them to put you in touch with someone who does.

Reiki is learned most often in a class with a Reiki Master. The class should consist of one to four Reiki attunements. During the class you should also be:
- shown how to give yourself and others Reiki treatments.
- given time to practice at least one self-treatment and one treatment on another person.
- told the five Reiki Principles and had time to discuss them.
- told the Reiki Story or Reiki history or both. Although the Reiki Story is not factual I like to tell it to my students because it is a metaphysical legend that helps you through your experiences of Reiki.
- given a background of Reiki, its terms, associated ideas and had the meaning of the word Reiki explained.

REIKI TERMS

Like other techniques Reiki has its own terminology.
Reiki
Reiki is a composite of two Japanese words, which are pronounced RAY KEY. To remind me how to say Reiki I think of it as the 'KEY that opens a RAY of energy'.

Rei means Spirit or Ghost. Mrs. Takata translated this word as universal. For me it means the spiritually guided knowingness of the universe—the energy that allows God to be in all places at once. This energy is all around us in limitless quantity and is available to help anyone who asks.

Ki means Life Force Energy. This is the energy that flows through all living things—humans, plants, birds, insects, animals and so on. It is what animates us and gives us life. When our Life Force is abundant we are healthy, strong and enjoy living.

Radiance Technique

This technique is also Reiki. Dr. Barbara Weber Ray, who was trained to Reiki Master level by Mrs. Hawayo Takata, founded this branch of Reiki and chose to give it an English name—Radiance Technique.

Eastern Reiki and Western Reiki

Since the discovery that the Gakkai (association) for Reiki practitioners that was set up by Mikao Usui in Japan in the 1920s still exists, the practice of Reiki has divided into Eastern and Western Reiki. Eastern Reiki refers to the Reiki techniques used by the Japanese Reiki practitioners who belong to the Usui Reiki Ryoho Gakkai and by those Reiki Masters whose lineages do not include Mrs. Hawayo Takata.

Western Reiki is the system that was taught by Mrs. Hawayo Takata when she introduced Reiki to the west. Today there are many Reiki practitioners who use both techniques.

Degrees

Reiki is traditionally taught as a number of degrees or levels. This is probably due to the fact that Reiki came from Japan where other disciplines such as karate are taught in degrees as well. Reiki has three degrees —1st, which is for beginners; 2nd, which is the next level; and 3rd, which is for Masters/Teachers. After Mrs. Takata's death several other degrees and a number of other classes have been added to Reiki that usually introduce the student to a variety of symbols and methods that can be used with Reiki.

Degrees of Reiki

Lineage

A Reiki lineage is the line of Reiki Masters who have passed Reiki along to you. My 1st Degree Lineage is: Mikao Usui, Chujiro Hayashi, Hawayo Takata, Barbara Ray, John Latz, Clarity Martin, Carrlyn Harring and Victoria Sinclair. In the West all Reiki lineages begin with the same three Masters—Mikao Usui, Chujiro Hayashi, Hawayo Takata. Mrs. Takata taught 22 people to be Reiki Masters and from each of them comes the lineages of Western Reiki.

Each lineage of Reiki differs in the way they teach Reiki because each Reiki Master has experienced Reiki slightly differently. No lineage is better or more important than another—just different.

As lineages get longer (more Reiki Masters between yourself and Mrs. Takata) the importance of knowing your lineage has diminished and today not everyone can tell you their complete lineage.

Reiki Practitioner

A person who has been attuned to Reiki, no matter what Degree, is known as a Reiki Practitioner. Once the practitioner is attuned to the universal life force energy it will flow whenever they place their hands on themselves or another person. The practitioner is not depleted of energy when they give a treatment because Reiki is channelled through them from beyond them. Reiki Practitioners benefit from giving others Reiki treatments because they also receive a healing as the energy passes through them to the receiver. Anyone can become a Reiki Practitioner because the universal life force energy benefits people of all ages, races, religions and intellects. To become a Reiki practitioner you have to be attuned to Reiki by a Reiki Master.

Reiki Master

A Reiki Master is a person who has completed 1st, 2nd and 3rd Degree Reiki and is able to teach and pass on Reiki to others. The way to activate the ability to do Reiki is by receiving an attunement from a Reiki Master. Usually the Reiki Master gives the student a hands-on attunement, which means the Reiki Master and student are in the same room so the Master can physically touch the student. Occasionally the attunement is done by the Reiki Master who lives some distance from the student and this is known as an absent attunement.

Each Reiki Master teaches Reiki their own way and each way is valid. Once you decide to become attuned to Reiki you will be drawn to the right Reiki Master for you.

Reiki Attunements

Reiki is transferred from Master to student by an attunement process. This process can be likened to radio waves that are all around us but can only be heard when a radio is turned on and 'tuned' into the radio frequency. An attunement is also called an initiation.

The attunement process creates a special link between the source of Reiki and the Practitioner. The source of Reiki is the infinite universal life force energy, not the Reiki Master giving the attunement. The Reiki Master facilitates the actions that create the link to Reiki. Once the attunement is completed, the Reiki Practitioner has his/her own direct link to the universal life force energy.

After you receive the First Degree Reiki attunement(s) you will have the ability to channel Reiki for the rest of your life. You can never lose that ability. Even it you don't use Reiki for a number of years it will still be there for you to use when you want and/or need it.

Religion or Belief

Reiki is not a religion. Nor is it a dogma or a belief system. You do not have to believe in Reiki nor do you need to fast or meditate for it to work. As easily as Reiki complements other healing therapies, it also complements religion because Reiki comes from God/Creator or Universe/Source (or whatever name you prefer). Using Reiki will increase your spiritual awareness and is likely to deepen your existing religious beliefs. It gives you a greater feeling of being in touch with a profound, healing and spiritual force that can only be described as the Creator or Source of all life. Reiki always works for good and can never harm. Reiki easily crosses all cultural and religious boundaries.

HOW REIKI WORKS

Channeling

A Reiki Practitioner acts as a conduit for the universal life force energy. The energy doesn't come from them but beyond them. Therefore a Reiki

Practitioner's energy is not depleted when they channel Reiki to themselves or someone else. Just as the inside of a drain pipe gets wet when it channels water, a Reiki Practitioner will receive some of the energy as it travels through them. This means that at the end of a Reiki treatment a Reiki Practitioner will feel energized and may have received a healing if it was needed.

Intent

The universal life force energy works co-operatively with the person channeling it. The practitioner can do this by using intent. An intent is a thought that directs or instructs Reiki to work on a particular issue. An intent tells the energy what you would like it to pay special attention to. As Reiki works for the highest good of the person receiving it, if your intent does not support the highest good of the receiver, Reiki will not activate your intent. This means the result of a Reiki treatment can differ from your intent. It also means that Reiki cannot be used for any negative intent or to harm anyone.

Before treating a person you can ask them what they would like Reiki to accomplish. This can be established at the time the appointment is made or just prior to giving a treatment. Once the person is comfortable and about to receive a treatment, place your hands on their shoulders and state the intent for the treatment—this can be done silently or aloud. For example:

Heal and bless Mary's knees. Ensure they are flexible and free of pain now.

Or you can use Mikao Usui's method of bringing your hands together in prayer and praying for the good health and well being of the person you are about to treat with Reiki. I have found Louise Hay's affirmations in her book *Heal Your Life* very useful as intents for Reiki treatments.

Intents increase in effectiveness when they are repeated at each hand position. This means it is best to keep your intents short, simple and easy to remember.

Don't worry if you forget to establish an intent or if the person you are treating doesn't want to use an intent. Reiki will still work although the person receiving the treatment may not necessarily begin their healing process in the area or way that they expected. The energy has a wisdom of its own and will always heal for the highest good.

Actions can contain intents. Just as a handshake contains the intent of friendship, the Reiki hand positions contain the intent of healing. If you place your hands in any of the Reiki hand positions without saying an intent the Reiki energy will still flow and heal.

You can also use an intent or affirmation while giving yourself a self-treatment.

Prayer

Instead of an intent you can start your Reiki Treatments on yourself and others with a short prayer. You can use a prayer similar to Mikao Usui's: *"I pray for the good health and well being of (say person's name) who is about to receive Reiki through me."* Or you can say your own prayer. Repeating the Lord's Prayer at each of the Reiki hand positions is another good way of adding more energy to your Reiki treatments.

Intuition

Reiki attunements have the ability to make you more aware of yourself, your surroundings and feelings. Because of this awareness you may find yourself becoming more intuitive. There is no need to be afraid of this. Learn to follow and trust your intuition and you will find yourself benefiting in many ways. Listening to your intuitive thoughts and feelings while giving a Reiki treatment will enhance your treatment and bring another dimension to your use of Reiki.

Intuition rarely comes as awe-inspiring revelations. It arrives quietly, almost tentatively, into your awareness. For me, my intuition has increased by small steps over the years I have been a Reiki Practitioner. It began as gut feelings and fleeting thoughts. Now, when I get into a car, I get a mental picture of the map of the whole route I am to travel and sometimes it is quite different from my usual route. I have learned to follow this map, which has often helped me to avoid traffic hold-ups. As I get out of bed in the morning I will have a feeling of wearing particular clothes and sometimes get a vision of the clothes to wear for the day. On several occasions I have been directed to wear casual clothes to work and then found that during the day I have had to do some very dusty, dirty work clearing out old files from forgotten cupboards.

Often I will know who is calling before I pick up the phone, or I will know the caller will be someone I have never spoken to before. When I get stuck with a problem I now ask Reiki for help and ideas begin to flow; they are often quite different from the usual or expected solutions.

The most effective way of making use of your intuition is to take notice of it. If you are given a picture of a different way to drive home from work then take that route and see what happens. If you have a thought to pick up something then pick it up. One day, when my mother, who is a 2nd Degree Reiki Practitioner, got to her bus stop she found a glass bottle broken on the footpath. She had a very strong urge to pick it up. And although she felt a bit silly she did pick it all up. As she was putting the last of the glass into a nearby bin two young men jogged by, one was barefooted.

Your intuition, I believe, is there to help you live your life better, safely, and with more joy, tolerance and ease.

Some Reiki Practitioners discover they have the ability to mentally see into the body. They find they can see the liver or kidneys, or find themselves travelling through the intestines or can observe the heart pump blood and so on while they are giving someone a Reiki Treatment. This ability has been called medical intuition. The author Carolyn Myss writes about this phenomenon in her books. She recommends that people who can do this, and want to know more about it, should study anatomy. Reiki Practitioners may also get smells or itchy noses while doing Reiki Treatments. I have found that a sour, stale urine smell indicates the person has a bladder or kidney infection, and a strong onion/metallic smell usually indicates the stomach is being affected by the medication the person is taking.

The different colors that people see in their mind's eye while giving a Reiki Treatment may also have specific meanings. I have found that a lot of red usually means an inflammation.

There is little or no information about these aspects of Reiki and the Reiki Practitioner has to observe, ask questions and keep a journal to build up a dossier of their experiences. Although you may get such information through your intuition it is not advisable that you use this information to diagnose a problem. Use the information instead to direct where you place your hands and how long you stay in that hand position.

Levels

We are made up of physical, mental/emotional (psychological) and spiritual levels. My understanding is that these levels are all of equal value—one level is not more important than another. Reiki works on all these levels to bring them into alignment and balance. These levels represent the different ways we operate in this world. The physical level includes our body, our actions and our speech. The mental/emotional level includes our thoughts, memories, ability to learn, intuition, talents, emotions and feelings. The spiritual level includes ideas, thoughts and feelings about God and the unknown, co-incidences and opportunities, auras, clairvoyance, life force energy, archetypes and symbols. Many Reiki Practitioners find they are drawn to the spiritual side of life, because this is a level that we do not usually pay a lot of attention to; and they focus less on their emotional level, becoming more relaxed, tolerant and balanced.

Processing

The release of toxins from the body is called 'processing' or 'the healing crisis'. These terms also cover the release of old ideas, old hurts, unwanted relationships, and so on. The more you do Reiki on yourself the more unwanted 'stuff' will be released. If you find yourself feeling out-of-sorts, maybe a little weepy or tired or things seem to be going wrong, it is highly likely you are releasing things that need to be let go of before a 'shift' can take place in your life.

Processing can occur as dreams, daydreams, return of old memories, dark depressing thoughts or moods and tears that have no explanation. When these happen you need to take some time to look at them and give permission for them to be released. Processing is the cleaning out of your physical, psychological and spiritual cupboards. Dreams and daydreams can be ways for Reiki to hold up an old memory, hurt, wish or feeling to see if you want to retain it, in the same way that you hold up an old dress or coat that has been sitting at the back of your closet to see if you still can fit it, if it is still useable and whether you still like it. If you no longer want or need the old memory, dream, wish or feeling then place your hands on yourself and mentally give Reiki permission to let it go from your life now.

Unexplained tears and moods, when you have no idea why you are moody or crying, I believe come from a time in your life when you had no words or ability to describe your hurt—when you were a baby or small child before you knew how to use language to describe what was happening to you.

To speed up the process and to make it easier to get through, drink plenty of water so that the unwanted toxins can be washed from your body as quickly as possible. Most importantly, keep giving yourself Reiki treatments. Once you have passed through this stage you will feel lighter, happier, healthier and more energetic.

Shifts

In the Reiki community we speak of the changes that take place in our lives as 'shifts'. Shifts can manifest as changes of attitudes, emotions and beliefs or they can be physical shifts—tiny jerks and twitches as parts of the body realign back into their correct positions. After having a Reiki attunement you may find your life undergoes a series of shifts as your body and all its levels become more balanced. This in turn will increase your energy and promote health in your life. Remember that Reiki is always working for your highest good. Although some shifts may seem insignificant or difficult or make no sense at the time they happen you will find, on looking back at your life, that they have all been for the best.

Scanning

Scanning is a process of sensing where a client needs more Reiki. Hold your left hand about one or two inches above the client's body (some people use both hands). While holding your hand(s) at that level slowly move them over the client's body. Notice what is happening with your hand(s)—are they getting warmer or tingling, pulsing or going cold? Those areas of the body where you feel a reaction in your hands are where the client needs extra Reiki. Take note of them and when you reach those areas during the Reiki treatment spend more time there or give those areas extra Reiki at the beginning or end of the treatment.

At first you may not notice much reaction in your hand(s) when you are scanning. The more you practice the more your scanning ability will improve. You can also scan yourself before a self-treatment.

During the scanning process you may feel lumps or feel your hands being blocked or stopped. When this happens stop scanning for a moment or two and hold your hands around the lump or over the block and allow Reiki to flow from your hands until you no longer feel the lump or block. Continue scanning.

Grounding

A Reiki treatment can sometimes make a client feel light-headed, slightly dizzy or sleepy. This can be overcome in several ways.

- Finish off the treatment by doing the Dry Bathing Technique (Ken Yoku) on yourself. This is the most effective method I have experienced for grounding both yourself and the client after a Reiki treatment. Although you do it on yourself it also has an effect on the client even though you don't touch the client during the technique.
- Give the client a glass of water to drink.
- Give the client an aura brush off—starting from the top of the client's head, holding your hands about about three or four inches above the client's body, move your hands in a circular brushing motion down their body from the head to their feet and back up to their head again. This will help the client to come 'awake' after the treatment. There are numerous ways of doing an aura brush off. If you are not sure which to use have a practice session with a couple of friends and try them all out until you find one you all agree feels right.

Support Groups/Exchange Groups

When Reiki Practitioners get together to give each other Reiki treatments, the meeting is called a Reiki Support Group or Reiki Exchange. These groups are highly recommended for Reiki Practitioners as they give you an opportunity to meet other Reiki Practitioners, to practice Reiki, talk about Reiki and speed up your own healing process while helping others with theirs. Your Reiki Master will probably know of a group in your area. If not, put out a request on one of the Reiki bulletin boards on the Internet or ask at your local health food store or New Age bookshop.

Monitoring/Reviewing

Many Reiki Masters allow you to sit in on the Reiki classes that you have already done. This is known as monitoring or reviewing. Usually there is no fee if you monitor/review a class with the Reiki Master who originally taught you, but a small fee if you monitor/review the class of a Reiki Master who has not taught you Reiki. Monitoring/reviewing a Reiki class lets you pick up information that you may have disregarded, dismissed or not understood during your first class. If you monitor/review 1st Degree Reiki, after several months of practice on yourself and others you will find you understand more and some parts of the class will become clearer and more interesting.

ENERGY EXCHANGE

The fee for a Reiki class or treatment is referred to as an Energy Exchange. There have been all sorts of theories about why there is an energy exchange for Reiki Classes. The example in the Reiki Story of Mikao Usui working with the beggars in Kyoto is often cited as the reason why there has to be a payment for teaching Reiki and for Reiki treatments.

For a Reiki Class

Most Reiki Masters have to pay for the cost of a venue, travel to and from the venue, manuals, morning/afternoon teas and sometimes lunch. For them to recover their costs and also to earn a living they need to charge a fee for teaching Reiki. If you do not agree with, or like, the fee a Reiki Master is charging for a Reiki class then look for another Reiki Master.

For a Reiki Treatment

By all means give your friends and relatives free Reiki treatments. When you first begin doing Reiki treatments the Energy Exchange they are giving you is the opportunity to practice and gain experience. However, as you become more experienced and you gain a reputation for using Reiki you will need to consider asking for an Energy Exchange. Some practitioners ask for a donation, some ask for a set fee, and others will accept vegetables or other goods in exchange. The choice is yours.

Many people feel happier if they can pay for their treatments in some way; it makes them feel in control of their healing and that they are also contributing to their wellness.

Don't Collect Debts

If you want to move into the higher realms when you pass on from this life do not collect debts. Don't owe anything to anyone and do not let others owe you anything, otherwise you will have to come back to this level of life again to either collect or pay your debts. This is what is known as karma. Doing Reiki without an exchange can set up a spiritual debt. You will know there is a debt when you have the feeling that a favor is owed either by you or to you.

THE REIKI STORY

The Reiki Story is the story Mrs. Hawayo Takata told about how Mikao Usui discovered Reiki. For many years this story was always told in every 1st Degree class.

The Reiki Story is not fact as many people in the West have discovered. For a while some people began to wonder if there really had been a person called Mikao Usui. Some Reiki Masters stopped teaching the Reiki Story in their 1st Degree classes. I still include the story in my classes because I believe it is a mythic story that gives us information on how to use Reiki.

Myths, legends and fairy tales are more than entertainment for children. On the surface they appeared to be stories about people, but on a deeper level they were also stories about how to live your life in a better way. This type of story is known as a mystical or esoteric story with hidden meanings that reveal themselves when the reader is ready.

The Reiki Story is very complex—containing within it several layers of meaning. The first layer, the one that we are most familiar with, is a simple story about how Mikao Usui discovered Reiki. However, because the Reiki Story is an esoteric story—a story with hidden meanings—it will unfold each time you read it and as you practice Reiki and progress through the degrees of Reiki. Because most of us are unfamiliar with the metaphysical concepts of Taoism and Buddhism the esoteric elements within the Reiki Story have remained hidden to Western practitioners of Reiki. My previous book, **Reiki and the Healing Buddha,** has an explanation of the esoteric aspects of the Reiki Story.

THE REIKI HISTORY

The history of Reiki is different than the Reiki Story. The history consists of the facts known about the three main people responsible for bringing Reiki to the West—Mikao Usui, Chujiro Hayashi, and Mrs. Hawayo Takata. The stories of these people and how Reiki made its way to the West can be found in the following books:

- *Living Reiki—Takata's Story* by Fran Brown
- *Hawayo Takata's Story* by Helen J. Haberly
- *Reiki Fire* and *Reiki—The Legacy of Dr. Usui* by Frank Arjava Petter

THE REIKI PRINCIPLES

Western Reiki Version	Eastern Reiki Version
Just for today, do not anger	*Just today*
Just for today, do not worry	*Don't get angry*
Honor your parents, teachers and elders	*Don't worry*
Earn your living honestly	*Show appreciation*
Show gratitude to all living beings	*Work hard (on yourself)*
	Be kind to others

Using the Reiki Principles

Whatever version of the Reiki Principles you prefer, they are to be used. They are not just fancy words to look at occasionally. Mikao Usui asked his students to actively work with the Reiki Principles by *'joining their hands together in prayer and praying to their heart and chanting the words with their mouth'*. Holding the hands together in prayer is an action with a built-in intent. It indicates that we are talking to God. This is not some god who is 'out there somewhere' but the 'God Within'. Saying the Reiki Principles while we hold our hands in prayer means we are speaking to the most sacred part of ourselves.

In my opinion the best way to the use the Reiki Principles is to add them to the Reiki treatments that you give to yourself and others. You can do this by silently repeating the Five Reiki Principles to yourself at each of the hand positions you use in a Reiki treatment. Done this way, the Principles are absorbed into the body, mind and spirit during a Reiki treatment and begin to work automatically in our lives without us having to make a conscious effort to use them.

The Meaning of the Reiki Principles

Each of the Reiki Principles will have their own meaning for you. Some of the principles have been changed over the years—often because people did not like or felt uncomfortable with the principles that were originally taught. If any of the principles challenge you it is probably because you need to do some work in that area. I was taught the Western version of the Reiki Principles that came through Mrs. Hawayo Takata's lineage and I still find them valid and useful in my life. My interpretation of these principles is:

Just for today, do not anger—this means that day by day you do not get angry, irritated or annoyed about anything or anyone. It isn't about being passive. It is about not getting angry. It means finding other ways of dealing with your problems. Anger often arises when we feel out of control or want to control something and cannot. Anger destroys relationships but it most often destroys the person who is angry. Anger tightens the blood vessels and makes the heart work faster and faster. People who regularly get angry are prone to heart attacks. Anger can act as a pointer to what thoughts and feelings you need to heal. Give yourself Reiki as soon as you notice your anger rising.

Just for today, do not worry—worry blocks ideas, solutions and also abundance. Let go of worry and the energy of the universe is able to flow into your life and activities easily. Worry causes lack of abundance, indecision and anxiety. Trying to stop worrying is easier said than done. I place my hands on myself and when the Reiki is flowing I ask Reiki to heal the problem I am worrying about. Then, whenever the problem returns to worry me I say to myself, *"Reiki is taking care of this."* This way I don't take it upon myself to solve the problem or worry about it. I hand it over to a higher power (Reiki) to take care of it. This has worked well for me.

Honor your parents, teachers and elders—this is about forgiveness. It is about rising up to your higher (honorable) self so that you can bless and forgive those who have hurt, angered, obstructed and censored you. Parents, teachers and elders are the hardest people in our lives to forgive. This principle is not about loving or obeying these people, it is about forgiveness. Once you have blessed them they are unable to hurt you anymore and you can let them go from your life. Thoughts about them will drop away and not arise.

Earn your living honestly—this is about being honest with your-self and how you are living your life. If you want to be happy are you doing something about it or are you just sitting around moaning? This principle will also help you to find what you really want to do with your life and help you to put your dreams into action.

Show gratitude to all living beings—this is about saying thank you to other people and other living beings as well as yourself. Do you appreciate you? When you have done something well do you accept the praise others give you or do you find fault with what you have done? Do you make excuses when someone gives you a compliment? Do you say thank you for your opportunities and good fortune? Do you praise and thank others?

Repeat these Five Reiki Principles at each hand position when you are giving yourself a Reiki Treatment and you will discover them working in your life without you having to consciously make them happen.

YOUR HANDS

Hygiene

Before and after a treatment wash your hands. Also take notice of how they smell. It is not pleasant for a receiver/client if they can smell onion, garlic, tobacco, or other strong odors on your hands, particularly when your hands are on their face.

You will not pick up someone's illness while giving them Reiki and they will not get any illness from you during a Reiki treatment. However, touch can spread infection so it does pay to take care of hygiene matters. If you are giving Reiki to an open wound or an infected area it is more hygienic for both yourself and the receiver/client to hold your hands an inch or two above the area or to place something between your hands and the infection/injury, such as a paper tissue or bandage.

The Sensations in Your Hands

During the course of a Reiki treatment Practitioners can experience a variety of sensations in their hands; heat which ranges from warm to very hot; tingling; cold; and pain, etc. *The Complete Reiki Handbook,* written by

German Reiki Master Walter Lübeck, provides a good description of the different sensations. In my experience:

Tingling generally indicates inflammation. The sides of my little fingers tingle like they have pins and needles when there is inflammation associated with arthritis. The palms of my hands tingle when there is a general inflammation and when I close my eyes I see the color red.

Cold—this happens where there is a long term problem that may have been around for years. When my hands go cold I leave them in that hand position until they feel warm again; this can take up to 20 minutes or more.

Pain—this pain is not the client's pain. As the person giving Reiki you cannot pick up the receiver's pain, ailments or problems. When your hands feel painful this means the area of the receiver's body is so negative no energy is able to penetrate it. Reiki needs to build up in your hands until the amount is greater than the negative/out of balance energy in the body. It is this build up of Reiki that causes the painful feeling. When Reiki is able to move into the receiver/client's body, your hands will stop feeling painful. The pain can be quite intense—sometimes building up into your arms and even as high as your shoulders. Don't flick the pain away. You will release the build up of Reiki and it will have to build up all over again because it still has to overcome the negative energy. Endure the pain until it releases of its own accord from your hands.

You may notice that the hand you use to operate a computer mouse can get painful. This is because the electricity within the mouse is negative energy and is preventing Reiki from flowing from your hand. When you place your hand on something Reiki will automatically flow, especially when it senses negative energy. Try not to leave your hand resting on a computer mouse when you are not using it.

Heat—the various intensities of heat that come from your hands indicate that Reiki is flowing as required by the receiver's body. The more you practice Reiki the hotter your hands will get because you are able to channel greater amounts of the energy. If someone has a recent injury your hands will often heat up very quickly. You may even sweat with the amount of energy you are channeling. If someone needs only a little or no energy, your hands may feel quite neutral. Sometimes a receiver/client's skepticism and tenseness at having their first Reiki treatment can block any sensations in your hands. It is always good to give more than one or two treatments because the more treatments a receiver/client has the more they will relax and begin to trust you and Reiki. Once they are relaxed they will begin to feel sensations in your hands and so will you.

Twitching—this occurs when a lot of energy is passing through the hands.

Finger moving—sometimes the fingers of a Reiki Practitioner will move of their own accord—tapping the area of the body receiving Reiki. I have noticed this happening with many Reiki Practitioners and am not sure why. At one support group, while receiving a Reiki treatment, my mind began having negative thoughts and a finger of the practitioner doing the hand positions on my head tapped my head. When I took my attention away from the unhappy thoughts it stopped tapping but when I turned my attention back to those unhappy thoughts the finger started tapping again. It was as though it was pointing out I should be more careful about what I was thinking; making me pay more attention to what I was thinking and being less automatic about it. It is possible that finger tapping points to an area of the body that is being affected by negative energy or thoughts and needs some attention.

Pushing Away Feeling—on several occasions I have experienced my hands being pushed away from the receiver's body. On one occasion it happened with a cancer patient who had decided a few days before to accept fate and let go of his will to live. His body 'pushed away' my hands when I tried to give him a treatment and no energy flowed from my hands. Frank Arjava Petter told me that whenever Mrs. Kojama, past president of the Usui Reiki Ryoho Gakkai in Japan and who had over sixty years Reiki experience, felt her hands being pushed away from a client she would tell him/her that Reiki was not the appropriate treatment and he/she should seek help from a medical practitioner.

No Energy—this can often cause doubt, surprise and bewilderment for Reiki Practitioners when no energy flows from their hands during a treatment. When it has occurred for me:

- The body did not require Reiki. One person had a perforated bowel. They had to have an operation to repair the damage. Another person had cancer and had decided they did not want to live any longer.
- The receiver believed she was incapable of receiving the life force energy and had held this belief for most of her life.
- It could indicate that your intent is not appropriate. I was asked to do Reiki on a young woman at work who complained of backache and overuse syndrome. I placed my hands on her spine and made the intent that Reiki would heal her back, neck and arms. Nothing happened.

I was aware I was showing off—trying to impress people by giving a Reiki treatment and had wanted an immediate miracle. I decided to step aside from my ego. Once I did so I received an intuitive thought that the pain she was experiencing had nothing to do with her back or overuse syndrome and she needed to see her doctor. She went to her doctor, who discovered she had a very bad infection in both kidneys.

As you work with Reiki you will build your own understanding of what your hands are saying when you experience different sensations. Keeping a journal or case notes of the treatments you give will help you to build your knowledge of how Reiki works for you.

USING REIKI

Once you have been attuned to Reiki you will have the ability to channel Reiki for the rest of your life. The more you use Reiki the stronger it will become and the faster it will flow.

On Yourself—21 Days of Self Treatments

One of the gifts of Reiki is being able to give yourself a Reiki Treatment. The Reiki Story tells us that each day for 21 days, while he was on top of the sacred mountain, Mikao Usui threw away a stone. A stone can represent those things in your life that weigh you down, block your pathway, or hurt you. It is recommended that you give yourself Reiki self-treatments each day for at least 21 days after your 1st Degree class. This allows your body, mind and spirit to integrate the Reiki attunement(s) that you received during your class and for the energy to begin the healing process within yourself on all levels. I discovered that after 21 days I had also established the habit of giving myself a Reiki treatment daily, which I have continued ever since.

The ideal self-treatment is to use all of the twelve hand positions and to hold your hands in each position for five minutes. However, doing a few of the hand positions or spending only a few minutes in each position is better than not giving yourself Reiki at all. You can give yourself Reiki with one hand or both while watching TV, talking on the phone, chatting to friends, waiting for an appointment, sitting in a meeting or doing other activities that leave one or both hands free.

Some people like to do their self-treatments at night in bed before falling asleep, some like to do them in the morning before getting out of bed, and others do them during the day while sitting in a chair or lying on the floor or on the bus or train going to and from work. Your choice of when and where to do self-treatments will depend on you and your lifestyle.

You can add the Five Reiki Principles to your self-treatments by saying them to yourself several times at each hand position. You can also have an intent with each treatment. You can use the 21 day program of intents that appear in *Reiki and the Healing Buddha* or use your own intents for what you want healed in your life, relationships, body, mind and spirit.

With Other Healing Therapies

Reiki will improve the effectiveness of other types of therapies including orthodox medical treatments. It will speed up recovery from surgery and injuries. If medicine is held between the hands and given Reiki it is believed Reiki will increase its effectiveness.

Many Shiatsu, Reflexology, cranial sacral, massage and beauty therapists have become Reiki attuned as it adds another dimension to these and other therapies that utilize touch and the use of hands. Reiki attuned therapists generally have warm hands when they do their work.

If you are ever asked to visualize energy coming through your hands, remember that you do Reiki and you do not need to visualize. All you need to do is place your hands where the energy is required. Here is a technique for losing weight that comes from Japan. It was originally known as the Crane Method and required a lot of visualization of energy flowing through your hands.

> *Place your right hand on your navel. Wait until you feel Reiki flowing. Then slowly move your hand around your abdomen in a clockwise spiral until you reach your sides. Stop, then begin moving your hand in a counter-clockwise spiral back in towards your navel. Stop and Reiki for a few minutes.*

Do this technique several times a day, especially after eating. It will bring your digestive system into balance. If you do this technique each day, after about three or four weeks you will notice an improvement in bowel movements and a loss of weight. However, emotional issues about eating can interfere with persevering with this technique.

On Animals

Reiki works on all living beings. Animals respond well to Reiki and they love the energy. I have found animals will come to you when they need a treatment and will often present the area they want treated. Follow your intuition when giving Reiki to animals. Be patient and calm. They will walk away when they have had enough.

Plants

Plants also respond well to Reiki. Remember, plants cannot live on Reiki alone. They also need to be watered.

- Before potting, Reiki the soil by holding your hands above it or on it.
- Hold plants and seeds in your hands and give them Reiki for a few minutes before planting.
- If the plant is already in a pot you can put your hands on the pot and intend that Reiki goes to the roots of the plant and from there to the rest of the plant or you can hold your hands above the plant and beam Reiki down onto its leaves.
- While sitting in your garden, hold your hands palms out and beam Reiki towards your garden. Try it for ten or fifteen minutes once a week and see how your garden responds. Because Reiki works on all living beings, including weeds and insects, use an intent such as 'for the health and well being of the rose plants'.
- Cut flowers will last longer if you give them a minute or two of Reiki each day. This can be done by either placing your hands on the vase or holding your hands an inch or two from the flowers and beaming Reiki at them.
- Reiki the fruit and vegetables you pick or buy to ensure they stay fresh longer.

Inanimate Objects

Reiki can be used on inanimate objects. In my experience the first effect of using Reiki on machinery is that it calms your feelings, fears and frustrations so that you can think about the problem more objectively. The next effect is that help often turns up unexpectedly.

For example, my car got a flat tire one night. Prior to using my car I had already placed my hands on my car and intended that it ran well and was protected from accidents and theft. When the flat tire happened I was able to stop under a street light so I had plenty of light to see. I sat for a moment and thought of Reiki and intended that Reiki would send me some help. I set my indicator lights on emergency flash and opened up the trunk to get out the jack (my father insisted I learn to change a tire before letting me get my driver's license). Within a minute or two a young man stopped to help. He discovered my spare tire was also flat and took it to the nearest garage to get it pumped up. He returned and changed the tire for me. All he would accept for helping me was my thanks. So, as he left, I silently intended that Reiki would ensure something really nice would happen in his life in the near future in exchange for helping me.

Car batteries can be recharged using Reiki. I personally have not had to do this. However, I was at a Reiki Support Group when one member excitedly told us that she had used Reiki to recharge her car battery. She placed her hands on the battery and intended that it be recharged. After approximately five minutes she started the car. She was thrilled to have had Reiki confirmed in this way. Unfortunately, once she got the car started she switched off the engine without running it long enough to ensure the battery stayed charged. She was unable to get it started a second time by using Reiki. So if you do start a car after doing Reiki on the battery remember to keep the motor running for a while to continue the recharging process. It has been suggested that Reiki softens the surface tension of the water in the battery to enable the chemicals to combine easily so that there is enough charge to start the car.

I had a car key jam in the lock of my car's gas cap. I wasn't able to turn the key or get the key out. I tried, and the service station attendant tried. We both used a lot of strength but just could not get the key out of the lock. Fortunately, I had a spare key in my purse so I was able to continue on my way to visit a friend who had just completed 1st Degree Reiki. I told her about my problem and showed her how I couldn't move the key. I said I would have to call a locksmith. She said she would try Reiki on it. I must admit I was very skeptical at the time. She held her hands over the key and gas cap for five minutes while we chatted. Then I tried the key again and it immediately came out of the lock. This seemed such a miracle to me that shortly thereafter I attended a 1st Degree Class to become Reiki attuned.

ABOUT REIKI TREATMENTS

Treatments versus Sessions

From time to time discussion arises as to whether giving Reiki should be called a Reiki Treatment or a Reiki Session. The choice of what to call giving Reiki is yours. A dictionary defines session as a sitting or meeting and a treatment as dealing with, or behavior to, a person or thing. Traditionally giving Reiki has been known as a Reiki Treatment. It has been called a Reiki Session by those who want to avoid giving the impression that Reiki can "treat" an illness or heal a particular problem, or by those who want to promote Reiki only as a relaxation technique.

Giving a Reiki Treatment

No matter who you give Reiki to, always treat that person as special. Give your Reiki treatment as professionally as you can. The ideal treatment consists of the receiver/client lying on a massage table receiving Reiki for approximately an hour. Place the massage table in a pleasant, quiet environment where you will not be disturbed. Take the phone off the hook or turn on your answering machine so you are not interrupted by calls. If you wish, play relaxing music during the treatment and maybe light a candle. Make the place where you give a treatment special and the treatment a special event.

- Let the receiver/client know how long the treatment will take. Tell them something about Reiki so they will feel at ease about having a treatment. A receiver/client remains fully clothed during a treatment; however, do suggest they wear loose, comfortable clothing for it.

- Ensure that both yourself and the receiver/client are comfortable.
  a. Make sure the massage table is the right height for you to use comfortably.
  b. Place a chair at the head and foot of the table so you can sit while doing Reiki on the head positions and the feet. Some practitioners

use a typist chair with wheels so they can push it around the table and remain seated throughout the whole treatment.

c. You may feel more comfortable when standing during a treatment if you take your shoes off.

d. Ask if they would like to use the toilet prior to the treatment because of the length of time it takes.

e. Ask the receiver/client to remove their shoes. They may also wish to remove restrictive items like ties, belts, jewelry and watches.

• Once the receiver/client is lying on their back on the table ensure they are comfortable.

a. Provide a pillow for their head.

b. Ask if they want some support under their knees. Place a small pillow or a rolled up towel under their knees.

c. Cover them with a light blanket or sheet.

• Ask if they have an intent for the treatment. This is optional. You may prefer to use your own prayer or not use an intent at all.

• Scan the aura for areas that may need extra time spent on them. Scanning is also optional—you may not feel comfortable doing this with some clients.

• Sit at the head of the table and state the intent (if there is one) either aloud or silently and then begin the Reiki treatment.

• Some receivers/clients will be quiet during the treatment. Others may want to talk. This does not mean using the treatment as a time to catch up on all the local gossip. Do that over a glass of water or cup of tea after the treatment. If the client wants to talk, let them and just be the listener. What they talk about will be part of their healing process; a way of releasing what has been disturbing their minds.

• When it is time for the receiver/client to turn over onto their stomach bring your request to do so gently to their attention and help them to turn over.

a. Take the blanket off them until they have turned over then cover them again when they have settled into place.

b. Change the pillow/support from under their knees to under their ankles.

- After completing the hand positions on their back, finish off the treatment by:
  a. Aura brush off then place one hand on their upper back and the other on their crown for a moment or two. Or, place one hand on the base of the spine and the other at the top of the spine for a moment or two. An aura brush off is optional if you do the Dry Bathing Technique on yourself.
  b. Tell the receiver/client the treatment is over, and that they should take their time sitting up and getting off the table.
  c. Do the Dry Bathing Technique on yourself. This is a wonderful technique that I cannot recommend enough. The more you use it the faster and stronger it works. The Japanese name for the Dry Bathing Technique is Ken Yoku.
  d. Give the receiver/client a glass of water.

The 'Do Nots' of Reiki

Most Reiki Practitioners have neither the training nor the experience to diagnose, suggest an outcome, or recommend giving up medication.

Do Not Diagnose—unless you are a registered medical doctor. Do not even try to diagnose what is wrong with the client. Just give them Reiki and know that the energy will heal in the best way for the client. If you feel worried about the client's health then suggest they visit their doctor—let him/her diagnose the problem.

If they have a problem that cannot be healed with Reiki your hands may be 'pushed' away from their body or Reiki won't flow. Suggest they visit their doctor. Don't frighten them—just say that Reiki doesn't seem to be the appropriate treatment for their problem.

Do Not Suggest an Outcome—Reiki always works for the highest and best interest of the person receiving it. That may not always be the outcome that the client or you expected. Reiki has a 'knowingness' that has a more far-reaching view than we have. What we think would be the ideal outcome may not be right in the long run for the receiver/client. Therefore the outcome is not your responsibility. You are responsible for channeling Reiki during the treatment.

Do Not Recommend Giving up Prescribed Medication—this decision must be made between the receiver/client and their medical practitioner and not by you. You can recommend they monitor their progress so they can discuss the matter with their doctor.

Unfortunately there are many people who have to take medication every day of their lives. Some people don't like doing that. They will try to maneuver you into giving them permission to go off their medication. Then, because they have passed the responsibility for going off their medication on to you, when things go wrong you will be blamed.

The Number of Treatments

Recommend to your receiver/client that they commit themselves to a minimum of ***three successive treatments*** within one week, regardless of why they are having Reiki treatments. Three treatments within a short space of time will allow for a rapid detoxification process (otherwise known as a healing crisis or processing). Little or no improvement may be apparent after one treatment but there is usually noticeable improvement after three. Most people have a need for more than three treatments. Discuss with the client whether they want to continue receiving treatments. You can then arrange to give them treatments on a weekly or monthly basis. If someone has a long-term problem, it is often best if they attend a 1st Degree Reiki class so they can continue their treatments themselves.

Length of Time for Each Hand Position

Five minutes spent on each of the 12 hand positions with two to five minutes on the knees and feet is ideal and will provide a treatment time of just over an hour. However, some Reiki is better than none so consider the circumstances and give the amount of Reiki that will fit within the timeframe the receiver/client and you have available.

Receiving a Reiki Treatment

During a Reiki treatment the receiver/client often snores and their reaction is to try to stop. Gently reassure your client that it is okay to snore—

everyone does, some more than others. When a person receives Reiki they often enter into three kinds of consciousness at one time.

1. ***Sleep Consciousness:*** Their body goes to sleep. This causes their breathing to change, which often results in snoring or other sounds as they breathe through their mouth. Because their body is asleep their throat is also asleep, therefore they may have little or no wish to respond to what is being said during the treatment.

2. ***Awake Consciousness:*** Their mind is awake and their hearing becomes more acute. They are aware they are snoring—they can hear themselves. They can also hear all the sounds in the room, which can often seem very loud and sometimes irritating. Sounds may seem louder during a Reiki Treatment, consequently many people prefer no talking and that music be played very softly during a treatment.

3. ***Dream Consciousness:*** Their attention is often focused on what is happening in their mind's eye (third eye) where they are observing colors or images—much like observing a dream.

When a receiver/client experiences a Reiki treatment in these three ways at once the Reiki treatment appears to work faster and more effectively. The receiver/client is more relaxed and has little or no resistance to receiving Reiki.

Client Records or Casebook

It is recommended that you keep some kind of record of the Reiki treatments you give. Keeping a record of treatments will build up your confidence in helping other people and also increase your knowledge and understanding of Reiki. Keeping notes about using Reiki and who you have given Reiki treatments to and the results of the treatments will benefit you—especially if you want to become a Reiki Teacher or if you work professionally as a Reiki therapist.

Remember that your records should be confidential and you should not discuss client names or their problems with others. Be as professional as possible in all your dealings with clients—regardless of whether they are friends, relatives or paying clients.

Maintaining records of the treatments you give will provide assistance if you apply for membership to organizations that require you to write case notes and provide evidence of the number of treatments you have given before you join them.

What to put in your case notes:
1. Name of person receiving a treatment.
2. Their address, phone and fax numbers, and email address.
3. Dates they receive a treatment.
4. How long the treatment took.
5. If you do more than one kind of healing modality, state which treatment you used. For example, massage, or massage and Reiki, or Reiki only or Reiki with Crystals, etc.
6. The reason why the client wanted the Reiki treatment. For example, a particular illness or injury, for stress release and relaxation, to try a Reiki treatment, etc.
7. Any results. Don't press anyone for results. Let them tell you what they have observed.

You can keep your case notes as a card index or filed in separate folders or in a notebook. If you use a notebook, number each page, use one page per person and index the book by writing a list of page numbers on the first page of the notebook and listing the name of the person beside the number that relates to their page.

Keeping a Journal

Keeping a journal will help you know more about yourself and Reiki. Note in it how Reiki is working for you, how you experience the Reiki in your hands, and what happens in your body when you are doing a self-treatment. Record in your journal when people compliment you on your health, the state of your skin, the amount of energy you have and how animals and children are attracted to you. See if the compliments come after you have been doing regular Reiki self-treatments. Record the shifts that occur in your lifestyle, attitudes and emotions.

Water

People giving and receiving Reiki should increase the amount of water they drink. The water will help the body eliminate the toxins released by Reiki. Begin by giving your receiver/client a glass of water immediately after their treatment and also drink some yourself. Each time you give someone else a Reiki treatment the energy is also working on your system, clearing out toxins. If you feel a little headachy either during or after a treatment this is often an indication that you need more fluid. Drinking a glass of water will usually clear the headache almost immediately.

You can enhance the water you drink by holding the glass in your hands and giving it Reiki for a minute or two. You can also do this to the water for animals and plants.

DOING REIKI TREATMENTS

The following are the ways I teach and practice Reiki treatments. They are not the only way Reiki treatments can be done. Open any book about Reiki and you will see that the traditional twelve hand positions can differ. Differences are okay. They seem to have come about because Reiki Practitioners often use Reiki intuitively rather than rigidly following a set of hand positions. The hand positions are guides to help you have the confidence to use Reiki on yourself and other people. If you don't receive any intuitive instructions on where to place your hands you know that you can give an excellent Reiki treatment by simply doing the hand positions you were taught in your 1st Degree Class.

The Hand Positions for A Self Treatment

Treating yourself with Reiki is an important element of the practice of Reiki. It is also one of the most valuable aspects of Reiki. Some natural healing methods are difficult to successfully practice on yourself. It is recommended that you get into a routine of giving yourself a daily Reiki treatment. It will not only heal any problems you may have but eventually it will help to protect you from getting ill.

The Four Head Positions

1. ***Eyes***—place your hands over your face with the palms of your hands covering your eyes and your fingers covering your forehead.
2. ***Temples or Ears***—slide your hands to the side of your head so the palms of your hands are over your temples. Alternatively, slide your hands so the palms of your hands are over your ears. Use whichever position feels comfortable.
3. ***Back of the Head***—slide your hands around to the back of your head so they lie sideways across the back of your head with your fin-

gertips pointing in opposite directions. The thumb of your lower hand will be across the base of your skull.

4. ***Throat***—slide your hands from the back of your head, along your jaw line, until the heels of your palms are together at the point of your chin. The smallest finger of each hand will be resting along your lower jaw.

The Four Front Positions

1. ***Chest***—place your hands flat on your chest with the fingertips just touching in the center of your chest.
2. ***Solar Plexus***—slide your hands down to your solar plexus—on the lower ribs just above the waistline.
3. ***Abdomen***—slide your hands, fingers still touching, down to your abdomen—just below the navel.
4. ***Groin***—place your hands along each groin, with the base of your palms on the hipbones and the fingertips almost at the pubic bone.

The Four Back Positions

1. ***Shoulders***—place your hands over your shoulders—fingertips just resting on the top of the spine and the outer edges of your palms close to your neck or where your hands feel comfortable.
2. ***Upper Back***—as this position is difficult to reach with both hands at once, place the palm of one hand on your chest and the back of the other hand behind you on your back (opposite the hand on your chest or as near as possible to opposite without straining). Reiki will flow through the backs of your hands, your fingertips, and through the palms of your hands. When half-way through the time you intend to spend on this position change your hands so that the hand that was on your chest is on your back and the hand that was on your back is on your chest. This relieves the tension on your arms and elbows.
3. ***Lower Back***—place your hands on your lower back with your wrists on your waistline and your fingertips pointing towards your legs. You can do this position with either your palms or the backs of your hands against your back—whichever is more comfortable for you.
4. ***Base of the Spine***—slide your hands down to the base of your spine. Place one hand over the top of the other. Once again you can use either your palms or the backs of your hands against your back—whichever is more comfortable for you.

Knees and Feet

Treating your own knees and feet can sometimes be uncomfortable or difficult. Reiki will flow to wherever it is needed and therefore will flow to your knees and feet, even if you only give Reiki to the upper part of your body. However, you can enhance the focus of Reiki by intentionally sending Reiki to your knees and feet. You can choose to:

1. Include in your initial intent that the energy will also flow to your knees and feet.
2. Beam Reiki to your knees and/or feet by holding your hands at a comfortable angle above your knees/feet and intend Reiki goes to them. This is a great way to practice directing Reiki to an area of the body without touching it.
3. Reiki your knees and feet as follows:

Sitting in a Chair

   a. Knees—place your hands over each of your kneecaps.
   b. Feet—lift one leg up and rest your ankle across the opposite knee so you can place both hands on either side of your foot. You may also like to spend time holding your ankle so that area also receives a direct Reiki treatment. Then do Reiki on your opposite foot.

Sitting on the Floor

   a. Knees—sit so your knees are bent and you can place your hands on your kneecaps.
   b. Feet—sit with your knees bent sideways and your feet in front of you. Either Reiki each foot separately by holding each one between both hands or place one hand on each foot so you Reiki both at the same time. You can also Reiki your ankles while sitting in this position.

Remember to always be comfortable. Being comfortable while you are doing Reiki ensures that you will enjoy using Reiki and you will keep on doing Reiki.

HAND POSITIONS WHEN GIVING REIKI TREATMENTS TO OTHERS

With Client on a Massage Table

The ideal Reiki treatment is to have the receiver/client lay comfortably on a massage table. This is the most comfortable position for both the giver and receiver. This treatment takes approximately an hour. You can spend 3 to 5 minutes in each hand position, depending on the time you have available to give a treatment. When you move your hands from one position to another move them one at a time. This means you will stay in contact with the client at all times during the treatment. The client will continue to feel the life force energy flow as you move about the table and will also feel secure about where you are and what you are doing while they have their eyes closed.

When buying a massage table ensure that the height of the table is right for you in relation to your height. If necessary get someone to lie on the table so you can see how comfortable your back and arms feel while giving a treatment. The height should suit you whether you are standing or sitting while giving a treatment. A table that allows space for you to put your legs under it while sitting at either end also ensures comfort.

The Four Head Positions

Make sure the receiver/client is laying comfortably on his/her back on the table as described previously. You can either sit or stand at the top of the table. Most Reiki Practitioners sit in a chair while doing the four head positions. Occasionally a practitioner feels more comfortable standing while doing these hand positions. This is often due to the height of the table.

1. ***Eyes***—resting your elbows on the corners of the table, put the heels of your palms on the receiver/client's forehead and your fingertips on their cheeks, so your hands cover their eyes. Curve your hands slightly so there is room for the receiver/client to blink. Allow space around the nostrils so the receiver/client can breathe easily. Alternatively hold your hands a few centimeters above the receiver/client's face so you do not touch them.
2. ***Side of the Head***—slide your hands to each side of the head. You can either cover their ears (good idea if they have indicated they have ear trouble), or place your hands on the side of their head (temple

area) in front of their ears with your thumbs lying across their fore-head. Use whichever position feels right for the client.

3. ***Back of the Head***—gently tilt their head to the left and place your right hand under their head. Tilt their head back onto your right hand. Place your left hand under their head. Allow their head to move until it is balanced comfortably in your hands. Your hands should feel comfortable to both you and the client. Your fingertips will be resting at the base of their skull, while the curve at the back of their head rests in your palms. When it is time to move from this hand position either push your hands down into the pillow and pull them from under the head or tilt the head first to one side then the other while taking your hands away, one at a time.

4. ***Throat***—place your hands in front of the client's throat, with your fingertips overlapping slightly at the point of the chin and your thumbs resting along their jaw line. Don't press against their throat. Reiki will move across the gap between your hands and their throat.

The Four Front Positions

You can continue sitting while doing the first hand position on the client's body. Remember that you will be leaning over the client's air space so hold your head to one side to avoid breathing their air. You can also stand up and move so you are standing alongside the client's torso.

1. ***Chest***—place your hands over the client's upper chest. If you are sitting your hands will be side by side with the fingertips pointing towards their toes. If you are standing alongside the client, your hands will be placed one in front of the other across their chest with the fingers of one hand under or close to the base of your other hand.

2. ***Solar Plexus***—if you have been standing alongside the client's body lift your hands, one at a time, from the chest area and place them onto the solar plexus. Never run or slide your hands across a client's body because most receivers/clients would find the movement objectionable. Always lift your hands, one at a time, when moving from one hand position to the next. If you have been sitting for the first hand position, you will need to get up and stand alongside the client. Place your hands one in front of the other with the fingers of one hand just under the base of your other hand across their solar plexus—on the lower part of the rib cage under the breast and above the waist.

3. **Abdomen**—place your hands, one at a time, across the abdomen area just below the waist.

4. **Groin**—place your hands along the groin area of the client's body. Hold your hands in opposite directions—near side: use your left hand and have the base of your palm on their hip bone and your fingertips on the top of the pubic bone; far side: use your right hand and have the base of your palm on the pubic bone and your finger tips on their hip bone.

Knees, Ankles and Feet

The knees, ankles and feet were not traditionally part of the original twelve hand positions but, because they are easy to reach when someone is lying on a table, they have since been incorporated into Reiki treatments. People often have long term problems with knees, ankles and feet so it is beneficial to give Reiki directly to these areas.

Knees—place your hands on their knee caps. Hold your hands there until the knees feel warm, or longer if there are any problems with the knees.

Ankles—place your hands on the top of their ankles. Hold your hands there until the ankles feel warm, or longer if there are any problems with the ankles.

Feet—move to the end of the table. If you have previously placed a chair here, sit down. Place your hands on the top of the receiver/client's feet until they feel warm. If you wish you can place your hands on the soles of their feet for a minute or two. This may feel awkward so use the backs of your hands for this position; they fit into the soles quite comfortably.

When I have finished giving Reiki to the receiver/client's feet I usually rub their feet for a moment or two. This brings their attention back to what you are doing. Then I ask them to turn over. See page 24 for a description of what to do as a client turns over.

The Four Back Positions

1. **Shoulders**—stand alongside the receiver/client's upper back. Place your hands across their shoulder blades on the upper back—one in front of the other with the fingers of one hand near the base of the other hand.

2. **Upper Back**—place your hands across the middle of the client's back, just above their waistline.
3. **Lower Back** —place your hands across the receiver/client's lower back, below their waist line.
4. **Bottom of the Spine**—place your hands, one on top of the other in a 'T' shape over the receiver/client's tailbone.
5. **Knees**—place your hands over the backs of the receiver/client's knees.
6. **Ankles**—place your hands over the backs of the receiver/client's ankles.
7. **Feet**—place your hands over the heels of the receiver/client's feet, then on their soles.

Client Sitting in a Chair

This treatment takes less time because you do not use all the Reiki hand positions. It is used when it is not convenient for the receiver/client to lie down. They may be in a wheel chair, have a back problem which makes lying down uncomfortable, they may not have time for a full treatment on a table, or a massage table may not be available. This way of doing a Reiki treatment is often used to demonstrate Reiki at fairs and health expos.

While giving someone Reiki in a chair remember to keep your arms and elbows relaxed and to stand with your feet slightly apart. Also stand so your body is not twisted. Always ensure you are comfortable while giving a treatment.

The Three Head Positions

1. **Eyes**—stand behind the receiver/client and place your hands over their eyes by resting the base of your palms on their temples in front of their ears with your fingers cupped over their eyes and the fingertips either almost touching or overlapping.
2. **Head**—stand beside the receiver/client and place one hand across their forehead and the other hand cupped across the base of their skull.
3. **Throat**—stand behind the receiver/client and place your hands around their throat with your fingers overlapping at the point of their chin and your thumbs resting along the jaw line. Don't press against their throat as that can cut off the client's ability to breathe.

The Four Body Positions

1. **Shoulders**—stand behind the receiver/client and place your hands lightly on their shoulders.
2. **Chest**—stand beside the receiver/client and place one hand over the upper chest area and the other hand opposite on their back ie: sandwich their upper torso between your hands.
3. **Solar Plexus**—move your hands down one at a time to the receiver/client's solar plexus—on the lower rib cage and above the waist line. Hold one hand on the front of the body and one on the back.
4. **Abdomen**—place one hand on the stomach area and the other hand on their lower back at the same height as the hand on their stomach. You may be more comfortable kneeling beside them for this position, or you may decide not to include this position in your treatment because you have to bend over to do it. Bending will make your back ache.

The Rest of the Body

Unless there is something specific that needs Reiki I finish the treatment at the abdomen. Don't bother to Reiki the client's groin as this area is not easy to access while they are sitting. I only treat the knees and feet if the receiver/client has indicated there are problems in these areas.

1. Sit on a chair and lift the client's leg up so it rests on your knees. Reiki their knee then foot. Then do the other leg the same way.
2. Sit or kneel alongside the receiver/client and place a hand on each knee. Then sit on the floor in front of the receiver/client's feet and put your hands on each foot.

Group Treatment

A receiver/client can receive Reiki from more than one practitioner at a time. If you are a Reiki Practitioner and you are receiving Reiki either from one practitioner or from a group you can also place your hands on yourself during the treatment and give yourself a self-treatment at the same time. Decide before the treatment how long it will take. If the entire group are Reiki Practitioners, take turns being the receiver.

With Two Practitioners—

on the front of the receiver/client

1. One person does the four head positions and the first body position.

2. The other person does the 2nd, 3rd and 4th body positions, the knees and feet.

This gives each practitioner five positions to do on the front of the body. Alternatively:

1. One person does the four head positions.
2. The other person does the four body positions.
3. Both can do the knees and feet while standing opposite each other with the receiver/client between them.

on the back of the receiver/client

The two practitioners can 'mirror' their hand positions down the back of the receiver/client. 'Mirror' means two practitioners stand one on either side of the massage table and place their hands opposite each other on the receiver/client so their fingertips are almost touching. They move from position to position in unison.

With Three Practitioners—

During a Reiki Support Group, when there are three practitioners to administer a Reiki treatment, sometimes the treatment is given only on the front of the receiver/client because there is less treatment time available. If the receiver is a client they would receive a treatment on both their front and back.

on the front of the receiver/client
1. One person does the four head positions.
2. One person does the four front positions.
3. One person does the knees, calves, ankles and feet.

on the back of the receiver/client
1. Two people do the four back positions standing opposite each other with the receiver/client in between.
2. The third person does the knees, calves, ankles and feet.

With a Large Group

If there are more than four practitioners (I have received Reiki from 12 people at one time) there is not much room around the receiver/client to move your hands to different positions or to follow the traditional 12 hand positions or even to follow your intuition. In such cases the Reiki Practitioners place their hands wherever there is a space on the body and they keep to that same position for the duration of the treatment. Usually, in large group sessions there is only time for a ten minute (or less) Reiki Treatment per person.

THE DRY BATHING TECHNIQUE

Finish off a treatment (both self treatments and on others) by doing the Dry Bathing Technique (Ken Yoku) on yourself. You do not need to do anything to the receiver/client. It seems to work almost like magic on the client. The receiver/client will open their eyes and be fully alert within a few seconds of you completing this technique on yourself. This is the most effective method I have experienced for grounding both yourself and the client after a Reiki treatment. I believe it is the missing element of Western Reiki.

a. *With your right hand:* stroke down your body from the top of your left shoulder across to your right hip.
b. *With your left hand:* stroke down your body from the top of your right shoulder across to your left hip.
c. *With your right hand:* stroke down your body from the top of your left shoulder across to your right hip.
d. *With your right hand:* stroke down your left arm—from shoulder to right off your fingertips.
e. *With your left hand:* stroke down your right arm—from shoulder to right off your fingertips.

The Dry Bathing Technique can also be used to disconnect after doing other natural healing modalities such as Massage, Reflexology, Metamorphic Technique, Shiatsu, etc. You can also use it to disconnect from negative thoughts and feelings that keep running around in your mind.

ENHANCING YOUR REIKI PRACTICE

Although there are a number of ways you can enhance Reiki at 1st Degree level you cannot manipulate Reiki for selfish or negative ends. First and foremost, Reiki works for the highest benefit of the person receiving it, not for the person giving it. The person receiving Reiki subconsciously decides how much or how little Reiki they will receive. Here are some reasons why you may want to make your Reiki practice stronger and suggestions on how to go about it.

I've given this person lots of Reiki and they aren't getting well. Sometimes the person receiving Reiki treatments wants to get well but is skeptical about the abilities of the person doing Reiki. Or, the person receiving Reiki treatments doesn't want to get well but likes receiving the attention and touch of a Reiki treatment. Or, the person doesn't believe anything will make them better, including Reiki. Or, the person has been sent by someone else and they are resentful about being made to come for a treatment.

The Reiki Story tells us about the young girl with a toothache—who had lots of excuses about why she couldn't get well (couldn't afford it—dentist lived too far away—etc). A toothache is hard to cure. Usually you have to go to a dentist and have the part of your tooth causing the pain taken out. The dentist does not cure your sweet diet or your excuses or the negative words you fill your mouth with, so sooner or later you get a toothache again.

In the Reiki story Mikao Usui asked for permission to put his hands on the young girl's face. It seems to me that although some people come along for a Reiki treatment they do not always give permission for the treatment. I have found there are three ways to deal with this.

1. Begin each of your Reiki treatments by holding your hands in prayer position and praying for the receiver's good health and well being (as Mikao Usui did), or
2. Just before you start the Reiki treatment you can ask the client to say out loud: *"I give permission for this Reiki treatment to heal me on all levels,"* or
3. Before starting the Reiki treatment place your hands on their shoulders and think to yourself *"This person has agreed to this treatment therefore they have given permission to receive Reiki for their highest good. This person's role is to allow Reiki to flow through them to heal them and my role is to be a strong clear channel for Reiki and to use Reiki in the best way I know how for their highest good."*

I want more energy to flow through my hands. You can ask for more energy to flow through your hands by asking Reiki to increase the energy flow by double, triple or multiples of five, ten or twelve. You can also increase the flow of Reiki simply by looking at your hands instead of looking off into the distance or closing your eyes. Some people enhance the flow of Reiki by using Tai Chi or Qi Gong techniques to move and increase energy. Also remember that the more you practice Reiki on yourself and others the stronger and quicker the flow of Reiki will be.

Can I use Reiki with other natural healing therapies?
Reiki works with all other forms of natural healing. Once you have been attuned to Reiki you will find it flows whenever you use a healing technique and whenever you have the intent to heal; especially those treatments where you use your hands such as Massage, Shiatsu, Magnetic healing and Spiritual healing. Reiki also helps with other techniques including counselling and hypnosis.

Can I ask Higher Beings to help with my Reiki Treatment?
Yes, you can ask Jesus Christ, The Virgin Mary, The Healing Buddha, Kuan Yin, the Bodhisattva Tara (who can heal 404 diseases), The Bodhisattvas of Sunlight and Moonlight (guardians of the Healing Energy) and angels and archangels to assist you when you give a Reiki Treatment. Place your hands together in prayer (Gassho in Japanese) and pray for their assistance during the treatment. Don't forget to thank them at the end of the treatment.

MY EXPERIENCE

The following are some of the ways that I recommend using Reiki (*they are based on my own personal experience and opinion and may not be the opinion or experience of other Reiki Practitioners or Reiki Masters*).

Arthritis—in my experience Reiki works well on arthritis. Give the receiver/client full Reiki treatments. When you come to the painful areas hold your hands there for at least ten minutes or more. Give at least three full treatments in the first week, then regular weekly treatments for at least six to eight weeks, then a treatment once a month for three to six months. I recommend that the receiver/client attends a 1st Degree Reiki class so they can also give themselves daily self treatments and that they also regularly exercise the area with arthritis. Reiki relieves pain, so the exercise should be free of pain.

Bacteria and Viruses—bacteria and viruses do not pack their bags and tiptoe quietly and considerately away from your body when you are attuned to Reiki. They leave kicking and screaming, forced out by your immune system. After several treatments, either self-treatments or from another person, you may come down with a cold or flu-like symptoms. Coughing, sneezing, releasing phlegm, shivering and fever are all ways in which the immune system rids the body of germs, bacteria and viruses. The aim of Reiki is to bring your body into balance, health and wellbeing and it will strengthen and activate your immune system to do this. The stronger your immune system the faster the body can rid itself of a whole range of germs and the quicker you will get over this activity, which is most often experienced as a heavy cold.

Bleeding—dress the wound with a bandage or sticking plaster then do Reiki on the area. If there is a lot of bleeding then apply pressure with your hands as well. If the wound is serious take the person to a doctor or call an ambulance. Small cuts can heal completely with twenty minutes or more of Reiki.

Blood Pressure—Reiki helps to bring blood pressure back into balance. While at a Health Expo at Dannevirke in 2000 a community health nurse set up her stand opposite our Reiki one. She gave those interested a blood pressure test and wrote the results down on a piece of paper to take away with them. One man had a test and then came to our stand. He asked what Reiki would do for him. I told him that it would reduce his blood pressure. He sat down for a 15 minute Reiki treatment after which he went back to the community nurse who tested his blood pressure again. Sure enough his blood pressure was considerably lower. She was so impressed she had a Reiki treatment too. I later found that blood pressure medication can sometimes interfere with this result. Reiki will clear the medication out of your system—making you feel well because you are no longer experiencing the side effects of the medication but it can mean your blood pressure will increase. You need to monitor your progress with a doctor so you can gradually reduce your medication and possibly go off it.

Broken Bones—have any broken bones treated by a doctor. Broken bones heal slowly and need to be set back into place so they heal straight. You can give the person with the broken bones Reiki until they reach a doctor. Reiki will not heal a broken bone before you get the person to a doctor but it will reduce pain, stress and inflammation. Before the bones are set it will probably be too painful to place your hands over the break. Instead place your hands on the person where it is most comfortable for you to reach—for instance their head, feet, solar plexus or abdomen areas. Once the bones are set and in plaster you can Reiki directly over the break. Reiki will work through a plaster cast. With regular Reiki treatments the bones will heal very quickly.

Burns—put the burn under running cold water until the area is cool. Then do Reiki on the burn. It is recommended that you don't touch the burned skin with your hands so that you do not introduce an infection to the area. Hold your hands a little above the burn and intend that Reiki heals the skin quickly and successfully. If the burn is serious see a doctor. Reiki treatments on burns usually ensure there are no scars.

Cancer—Reiki doesn't cure cancer. Cancer is a parasitic entity of cells, which (as cancer) are healthy, and do what cancer cells do. It is the effect of the cancer on the body that is the problem. As the cancer grows it begins to destroy the body and becomes life threatening when it grows on a vital organ or becomes so widespread the body can no longer function. Cancer has to be killed and Reiki does not kill. At present cancer, if caught early enough, is most effectively treated by drugs, surgery, chemotherapy and radiotherapy. Reiki can assist by helping the body to quickly return to normal after surgery, chemotherapy and radiotherapy. Reiki enhances the immune system whose job it is to protect the body from illness.

Colds and Flu—in my experience the longer you use Reiki the less likely you are to catch colds and flu because regular use of Reiki seems to strengthen the immune system. If you do catch a cold you will not have it as long as non-Reiki people do. If you give yourself Reiki treatments for at least an hour each day you will usually get over the cold in a few days. Being attuned to Reiki does not mean you will never get a cold. I believe a cold is one of the body's methods of housekeeping; a way of cleansing the body of germs.

Depression—most people feel like smiling after a Reiki treatment. It lifts their spirits and relieves depression. It will often bring out the problem that is causing the depression in a way that the client can handle easily or the problem will simply disappear and no longer be a problem. Attitudes will become more flexible and daily living will seem easier to cope with.

Dying—Reiki helps with the process of dying. It relieves pain and stress and helps the dying to accept what is happening. It allows a person to die peacefully. It is my belief that the more peacefully we die the more fortunate the journey beyond death will be.

Fever—a high temperature is one way the immune system kills bacteria and viruses. If you are doing a Reiki treatment on someone who has a fever you may find their fever gets worse and as they get hotter they can get a very painful headache. This headache means the brain is getting dehydrated. You will need to let the person sip water regularly during the treatment. Sometimes the fever will break (they start sweating) during the treatment—make sure they do not get cold; ensure they are warmly covered. Sometimes the fever breaks after the treatment while they are sleeping. Reiki treatments do not stop a fever but appear to speed up the natural progress of a fever so the receiver/client gets through it faster.

Flying—if you experience discomfort in your ears during descent place your hands over your ears until the pain clears. If you feel air sick place one hand on your solar plexus and the other hand at your back opposite your solar plexus. Your body's balance mechanism is in your ears. Air sickness is caused by feeling out of balance, so also do Reiki on your ears. In both instances intend that you are balanced and safe.

Injuries—do any First Aid that is required, then Reiki. Get an ambulance or take the person to a doctor if serious. Reiki works quickly on new injuries. In my experience a recent injury will draw through a lot of energy and I have often broken out into a sweat because of the amount of energy passing through me. The injury will heal quickly and leave little or no scars. Injuries that have happened some time in the past take longer to heal as Reiki needs to also heal the mental, emotional and spiritual levels of the injury as the older an injury is the more time it has had to permeate through all levels of the body. Torn ligaments and tendons also take a while to heal, often because they are in places where there are few blood vessels (blood transports the immune system to the place of injury).

Lumps—in the glands and breasts, in my experience, respond well to Reiki. Simply place your hands over the lump several times a day and Reiki for as long as possible. If you are treating someone else, hold your hands over the lump for ten or more minutes during a full treatment. If the lump is in the breast ensure you have the permission of the receiver/client to place your hands on their breast, otherwise hold your hands one or two inches in the air above the breast—Reiki will still flow to the area it is needed. If the lump does not dissolve after three treatments over three consecutive days or less, see a doctor.

Motion Sickness—place one hand on your solar plexus and the other hand on your back opposite your solar plexus. Give yourself the intent that you are in balance. Also give Reiki to your ears.

Pain—place your hands directly over the pain. Reiki will diminish pain quickly. However, pain usually indicates that something is out of balance in the body. If the pain has recently appeared, it is advisable for the person to see their doctor for a check up. If the person has already seen a doctor about the pain, recommend they receive three full treatments in one week with follow up treatments once a week until the pain no longer returns. If the pain is chronic—ie: it has been around for a long time—recommend the person attend a 1st Degree Reiki class so they can give themselves full Reiki self treatments daily. They will then be able to Reiki the specific area whenever the pain occurs.

Menstrual Pains—regular Reiki treatments will diminish menstrual pains. I would recommend you attend a 1st Degree Reiki class as it is more convenient to give yourself Reiki treatments during your menstruation. I personally feel that Reiki works first in the reproductive area. You will find, with regular Reiki treatments, that each month your menstruation will become more normal and pain free. The hand positions for the head, throat, abdomen and groin all have an effect on the reproductive system of the body.

Pregnancy—if you are having trouble conceiving a child I recommend that both parents receive Reiki treatments and also become attuned to Reiki.

Continue with self-treatments throughout the pregnancy. I have observed that Reiki often works first of all in the reproductive areas—after all it is a LIFE force energy and therefore a major aim of the energy is not only to benefit life but support it in regenerating. Mrs. Takata apparently had a great deal of success treating childless couples.

Giving Reiki to a pregnant woman is both safe and beneficial for both her and the baby. Reiki treatments after the birth of a baby will speed recovery, relieve stress and post natal depression, and enable the mother to cope with a newborn baby. It also seems to assist with the birth process so that it is not as painful, long or complicated.

Relaxation—Reiki is ideal for dealing with stress and helping you to relax. A Reiki treatment is as relaxing as a massage. Some people relax so much they drop off to sleep during a treatment. Relaxation is the first step to healing.

Singing—since becoming attuned I have noticed a big improvement in my voice. The tone and range have improved. Reiki hand positions on the face, throat and chest help to improve resonance, tone and breathing.

CONCLUSION

The first rule of using Reiki is, I believe, to use your common sense. Don't throw out all your tried and true remedies and replace them all with Reiki. As a healing technique, Reiki works very well in conjunction with all other healing therapies.

The best recommendation I can give is practice, practice, practice. The more Reiki you do on yourself and others the faster and stronger it will flow and the more you will benefit in your own health and well being.

The hidden gift of Reiki is courage. It gives you the courage to change, to discover who you really are, to follow your dreams, to believe in yourself and to accept yourself with compassion.

The hidden lesson of 1st Degree Reiki is to learn to be non-judgmental about yourself, others, and the world around you. It helps us to accept that the mistakes we make are simply part of learning. Being non-judgmental of yourself and others is the first step to self-acceptance and self-compassion. Whenever you judge someone else you are also judging yourself. Reiki does not judge. It is available to everyone without prejudice

RECOMMENDED READING

There are now lots of books about Reiki and natural healing available for sale and from libraries. Here are just a few that I found interesting and helpful in understanding the energy, the history, and healing.

The following books look at the history of the people who brought Reiki to us—Mikao Usui, Chujiro Hayashi and Mrs. Hawayo Takata.

Fran Brown. *Living Reiki—Takata's Teachings*. USA: LifeRhythm, PO Box 806, Mendocino, CA 95460, USA

Helen J. Haberly. *Hawayo Takata's Story*. USA: Archidigm Publications, Garrett Park, USA

Frank Arjava Petter. *Reiki Fire*. USA: Lotus Press, PO Box 325, Twin Lakes, WI 53181, USA

The following books look at Reiki and using Reiki. There are many other books available that are equally as good.

Bodo J. Baginski and Shalila Sharamon. *Reiki Universal Life Energy*. USA: LifeRhythm, PO Box 806, Mendocino, CA 95460, USA

Klaudia Hochhuth. *Practical Guide to Reiki an Ancient Healing Art*. Australia: Gemcraft Books, 291-293 Wattletree Road, East Malvern, Victoria 3145, Australia

William L. Rand. *Reiki The Healing Touch*. USA: Vision Publications, 29209 Northwestern Hwy, #592 Southfield, MI 48034, USA

Walter Lübeck. *The Complete Reiki Handbook*. USA: . USA: Lotus Press, PO Box 325, Twin Lakes, WI 53181, USA

The following books look at the mental/emotional and spiritual reasons why the body is not well. They are also useful as a source of affirmations and intents.

Louise L. Hay. *Heal Your Life*. USA: Hay House Inc, 501 Santa Monica Boulevard, Santa Monica, CA 90401.

Annette Noontil. *The Body is the Barometer of the Soul*. Australia: Annette Noontil, Box 296, Nunawading, Victoria 3131, Australia

Debbie Shapiro. *Your Body Speaks Your Mind.* Judy Piatkus (Publishers) Ltd., Windmill St., London W1P 1HF, 1996.

I believe the Light seen in a near death experience is the source of Reiki. The following book looks at near death experiences and the healing aspect of the Light.

Kenneth Ring and Eveylyn Elsaesser Valarino. *Lessons from the Light— What we can Learn from the Near-Death Experience*. Insight Books, Division of Plenum Publishing Corporation, 233 Spring St, New York, NY 10013, USA. 1998.

The following books provide an insight into medical intuition and healing.

Caroline Myss. *Anatomy of the Spirit*. Bantam Books, 1997.

Caroline Myss. *Why People Don't Heal and How They Can*. Bantam Books, 1997.

Chapter Two...

2nd Degree Reiki

A journey is enhanced by the company you keep.

May you travel along the path of light and healing

In grateful and happy companionship

With the protection, compassion and wisdom

of the Reiki Symbols

ACKNOWLEDGEMENTS

*M*y thanks go to Reiki Master Bobbe Free, my 2nd Degree Reiki Teacher, to Reiki Masters Lynne Walker, Nigel Chan and Tina Webb for inviting me to monitor their 2nd Degree Reiki classes, to Reiki Master Elizabeth Currey for including me in her 2nd Degree Review class, to Reiki Masters Randall Hayward and Margaret Underwood for their 2nd Degree Advance classes, to all the Reiki Practitioners who attended my 2nd Degree Support Group, and to all my 2nd Degree Reiki students who opened my eyes to the infinite variety of 2nd Degree Reiki.

WHEN TO LEARN 2ND DEGREE REIKI

It is the student's choice when to learn 2nd Degree Reiki and they should not be coerced or pressured by others to do this degree before they feel ready. Traditionally it was recommended that a student spend about three months or more practicing 1st Degree Reiki before moving on to 2nd Degree. Some Masters ask that the student does 21 days of self treatments before they attend a 2nd Degree class.

Traditional Reiki Masters usually give four attunements during their 1st Degree classes that have a profound effect and need some time to integrate within all levels of the student. Today there are Reiki Masters who will accept and sometimes expect their students to do their 2nd Degree training the same weekend they do their 1st Degree class. However, these Reiki Masters usually give only one attunement at 1st Degree so the impact is not the same as receiving four attunements and less integration time is required.

As a Reiki student you should never feel obligated or pressured to do your 2nd Degree class with the same Reiki Master who taught you 1st Degree Reiki. It is your choice whose class you attend. Choose a Reiki Master whose personality and style of teaching suits you. It is easier to accept instructions from a teacher you like and respect.

Each Reiki Master teaches the 2nd Degree class of Reiki based on the experience of their lineage. The basics are usually similar. Perhaps the biggest difference is in how the Reiki Master draws the symbols that are taught during a 2nd Degree class. Because your Master is the "right Reiki Master for you" the way they teach the symbols is also right for you. Later you may feel you need to relearn the drawing of the symbols and that will be right as well.

Recommendation

If you learned the Power Symbol during your 1st Degree Reiki class, make sure your Reiki Master activates the Power Symbol again during your 2nd Degree class. At the first level of Reiki the Power Symbol simply protects—it does this for all Reiki Practitioners whether they have been taught to use the symbol or not. Symbols are said to "sit in repose" at the first level where they promise to protect all those who use the healing energy. During a 2nd Degree class the symbols are activated so they do infinitely more than just protect you when you use them.

If you have already done a 1st and 2nd Degree class where the Power Symbol was activated at 1st Degree but not at 2nd Degree, go back to your Reiki Master and ask that the symbol be activated in a 2nd Degree attunement. This is an important and necessary aspect of 2nd Degree Reiki and one to which, I believe, every Reiki student is entitled.

THE SECOND LEVEL OF REIKI

Content

A 2nd Degree Reiki class will give you a basic understanding of the first three Reiki symbols and how to use them. You will then gain an even greater understanding of the symbols as you use them, experience them and experiment with them each day.

It is important to learn how to both speak and draw the symbols because the universal life force energy responds to their sound and imagery. You need to know how to draw the symbols on paper, in the air, in your mind's eye or simply visualize them so that you can use them no matter where you are or what you are doing.

As you become more familiar with these symbols, by using them daily, you may notice that there will often be variations in the way you draw the symbols. You may find that the symbols will differ depending on the person, situation or goal that you are working with. This is due to the "wisdom of the energy." The symbols appear to reflect the healing that is needed at the time they are drawn for that particular person or situation.

WHAT ARE SYMBOLS?

A characteristic of a symbol is that it can express many meanings simultaneously and on different levels. There are three kinds of symbols:

1. **A physical representation.** This is the actual physical manifestation of something. For instance: water—on the physical level it keeps life alive on this planet. Water is also a symbol for all that keeps us alive, for example, money and the life force energy. This idea of physical things being able to represent abstract ideas is found within the art of Feng Shui.

2. **A personified representation.** This is when the physical article is represented as a human being. For instance: water—the ocean is represented by Neptune and the Oceanides (daughters of the ocean), and the rivers and streams by Naiads (fresh water nymphs). Many wells in Europe are sacred because they are associated with a goddess or saint. This level is associated with our inner need to define the world by human characteristics. This level of a symbol allows us to describe emotions, energies and ideas in the same way we describe people. These symbols have the power to provoke emotions and to modify our emotions.

3. **A letter of a sacred alphabet**. Some of the earliest written languages were developed to receive messages from God; for example, the Runes of Scandinavia, the Ogram of the Celts, Sanskrit of India and Chinese calligraphy. Alphabets and written characters let us describe an abstract idea. This is the most profound use of symbols. These symbols can reach a level of consciousness within us that we cannot define in other terms because it is beyond our interpretation. These symbols have the power to elicit the unknown into recognition.

THE REIKI SYMBOLS

The Reiki symbols and the Universal Life Force Energy operate at a level and a dimension that is much higher than the level on which we exist. Therefore they have a very expansive overview of what is happening and will happen in our lives. They operate for our highest good, which means that shifts and healing take place in our lives in unexpected ways —not necessarily how we envisage or intend they should. Reiki energy and the Reiki symbols always heal by creating changes and shifts for our highest good.

There are differing opinions about where the Reiki symbols came from. The story, as told by Mrs. Takata, tells of Mikao Usui learning about the symbols during a spiritual experience of oneness with the Pure Light Energy on the mountain of Kurama after meditating for 21 days. He saw beautiful colored bubbles containing the symbols. Others say Chujiro Hayashi added the symbols into the Reiki system after Mikao Usui's death.

I believe that whoever added the symbols into the Reiki system is not important; they work and have a profound effect on our lives. Paul Tillich, writer of *On Art and Architecture*, says that symbols come out of the depths of our soul to reveal realms of existence that cannot appear to us in any other way and that we cannot intentionally produce them.

There is a train of thought within the Reiki community that we don't need the Reiki symbols. Members of the Reiki Gakkai (Reiki Association) in Japan apparently do not use symbols and this has some people believing they don't need to bother practicing them or using them—preferring to use intent instead, which gets stronger, quicker and more effective as we continue our practice of Reiki. For me the symbols are an amazing gift that benefit everyone who makes a commitment to journey along the Reiki pathway at the 2nd Degree level. We are very lucky, and I am grateful, that they have been included in the system of Reiki that was initially taught in the West.

Sacredness and Secrecy

In the past the Reiki symbols were treated as both sacred and secret. That secrecy no longer exists. The Reiki symbols can be found in books and on the Internet. This does not diminish their effectiveness or their sacredness. These symbols do not work until you have received an attunement/initiation, which empowers and activates the symbols. Once you have received the attunement the symbols will work every time you use them.

I believe that initially it was the second level itself that was secret, not the symbols. The second level is the mental/emotional level of Reiki. Only you know what goes on inside your mind and heart. Another person can only guess at what your thoughts and feelings are. Until you choose to express your thoughts and emotions as words they are your secret.

The Reiki symbols are sacred because they represent an aspect of the creative power of the universe that we call God or know as God, and may contain a name of God within them. In the past the true name of God was rarely used—letters, symbols, images and numbers were substituted to represent God.

Each of the Reiki symbols is associated with a Buddhist deity. They are the essence or seed symbol (bija) of Bodhisattvas (enlightened beings who have promised to help humanity reach enlightenment). This does not mean you need to believe in Buddhism or that you have to become a Buddhist. A Buddhist deity is just one way of representing God, or the energy of the universe that has an effect on us, and our lives. Many Buddhist deities have found their way into Buddhism from far older religions because they represent a basic truth of life and spirituality.

Composition of the Symbols

Each symbol has a Japanese name, a translation of that name, an English name and a "pledge" or intent. Although you can use any intent with each symbol your intent does not override the original intent of the symbol. If your intent contradicts or does not support the original intent of the symbol it will not be acted upon.

JAPANESE NAME	TRANSLATION	ENGLISH NAME	INTENT	LEVEL WITHIN 2ND DEGREE
Cho Ku Rei	Imperial Edict, or Royal Command	Power Symbol	Put the Power of the Universe here	Physical
Sei Hei Ki	Sound together Wood	Mental/ Emotional Symbol	God and Humanity become One	Mental/ Emotional Level
Hon Sha Ze Sho Nen	Book (This) Person Righteously Corrects Thoughts	Distance Symbol	The Buddha in me reaches out to the Buddha in you in Peace and Enlightenment	Spiritual level

The symbol is a picture of the energy. This picture seems to indicate what energy is to be activated. The Japanese name of the symbol is associated with the sound of the energy and indicates how the energy is to be used. The Universal Life Force Energy (Reiki) appears to interact with the image and sound of the symbol to activate the intent of the symbol.

When I use a Reiki symbol I draw it once and speak or think its Japanese name three times. This is the way I was taught to use the symbols. This practice has become a habit of mine. Other Reiki Practitioners say the

Japanese name up to seven times and some only say it once. Each way seems to work well.

Drawing the Reiki Symbols

Reiki was discovered in Japan, therefore the method for drawing the Reiki symbols is based on drawing Chinese and Japanese characters. This method particularly applies to the Distance Symbol because it is a set of Kanji characters. Kanji is the name for the formal written language of Japan, which originally came from China. A Kanji character is meant to appear the same way each time it is drawn. The following are the basic rules for drawing Kanji that are traditionally taught within the system of Reiki for drawing Reiki symbols.

1. Draw the horizontal lines before the vertical lines.
2. Draw the horizontal lines from left to right.
3. Draw the vertical lines from top to bottom.
4. Draw a left stroke before a right stroke.
5. The exception to drawing a left stroke first happens when a right or middle stroke is longer than the left stroke. The longer or "elder" stroke is drawn first before any shorter or "younger" strokes; in other words, "elders first".
6. Any strokes that create a 7 shape are drawn as one stroke, starting from the outer edge of the horizontal stroke, regardless of whether the vertical part of the stroke is straight or curved.
7. When you draw a box shape with a stroke inside it, draw the left side of the box first from top to bottom, the top and right sides of the box are drawn next as one stroke. Then the stroke that goes in the middle of the box in drawn next. Finally the bottom line of the box is drawn.

The Order of the Reiki Symbols

The three Reiki symbols are taught in order from the simple image to the complicated image; ie: the Power Symbol first, Mental/Emotional Symbol second and Distance Symbol third. This allows you to get used to the symbols. The symbols are sometimes referred to as No. 1 (Power Symbol), No. 2 (Mental/Emotional Symbol), No. 3 (Distance Symbol); based on the order they are taught.

The Reiki Symbols can be used in any order. Their order of use seems to direct the focus of Reiki. The first symbol used will be the first focus of the energy. You can use a symbol on its own or two of them together or all three.

You can use one symbol or several by either choosing a random number or you can ask your intuition how many symbols you need. ***Draw the symbol you have chosen and say its Japanese name, then mentally ask yourself for the number you have chosen, or been given, of the symbols to do, whatever it is you want them to do.*** For instance you can ask that 20 Power Symbols clear and cleanse your liver or 100 Power Symbols protect your house or 1,000 Mental/Emotional symbols clear away all the negative thoughts and feelings from your street after someone has had a fight in it.

I was once asked why I use more than one symbol at a time. This was something I was taught to do by American Reiki Master, Randall Hayward, when he visited New Zealand. I have since worked with this method a lot and found it very effective. Often I ask my intuition how many symbols to use in a particular instance and the answer is usually more than one, sometimes it is under 20 and other times it is more than 100. I believe using more than one of the same symbol at a time is similar to Buddhists using sixteen vajras to surround a mandala or having a deity that has a thousand hands.

THE POWER SYMBOL

The Power Symbol is based on a counter-clockwise spiral. The clockwise spiral represents the journey of the sun. The counter-clockwise spiral is associated with the journey of the moon. As the practice of moon worship was replaced by other religions, anything associated with the moon became a sin. Sin is an ancient (Babylonian/Assyrian) name for the Moon. Consequently the counter-clockwise spiral has been out of favor for a long time. In all cultures around the world people have drawn spirals—both clockwise and counter-clockwise. In the East the counter-clockwise spiral is said to bring blessings and good fortune. The spiral is one of the building blocks of life and can be seen in the way sea shells and snail shells are formed and in the unfurling of ferns. The cells in our bodies form in counter-clockwise spirals.

The Power Symbol has nothing to do with how energy flows on Earth in the Northern and Southern Hemispheres. It remains a counter-clockwise spiral regardless of where you live. It is not an earth energy—it is an energy of the sky/universe. The Power Symbol represents a thunderbolt, which is a sky energy.

As you experience the energy of the spiral you will begin to be more aware of it in your environment. I have noticed that companies that use the counter-clockwise spiral in their logos are often very successful. Dr. Who, a long running TV program about time and space, used a counter-clockwise spiral as a graphic interlude between scenes.

Origin of the Power Symbol

The Power Symbol is the essence or bija (seed symbol) of the Bodhisattva Vajrapani; a fiery bodhisattva of protection. The word Vajra means Thunderbolt. Buddhism took the Vajra from the thunderbolt held by the Hindu god, Indra. Thunderbolts were held by many of the early gods of various civilizations. The Gods of Rome and Greece, Zeus, Mercury and Jupiter, all carried thunderbolts. The Christian/Hebrew God was also known to be associated with the thunderbolt—there is an old belief that if you did something to upset God you were liable to be struck by lightning.

In Buddhism the Vajra is also a symbol of wisdom with power over illusion and evil spirits (negative thoughts). It is believed to have the qualities of both the diamond (indestructible energy) and the thunderbolt. In its association with healing (The Healing Buddha mandala) the Vajra has three levels. At the first level it is known as a Yaksha General who has promised to protect all those who use the Healing Energy. This happens automatically during the 1st Degree attunement(s). At the second level, when the Power Symbol is activated during the 2nd Degree attunement, the vajra becomes a Bodhisattva known as Vajrapani (Thunderbolt in the hands). As a Bodhisattva (an enlightened being) he promised to help humanity reach enlightenment. At the third level, during the 3rd Degree attunement, the Vajra becomes known as Vajradhara (Thunderbolt King). He promises to bless you with whatever you wish, intend or focus your thoughts on.

What the Power Symbol Does

The Power Symbol can be used in all kinds of situations. My suggestion is that if you don't know which symbol to use, try the Power Symbol and see what happens. Some results will happen quickly and others will take a little longer. The more you use the symbols the quicker the energy and the results will be.

A Thunderbolt

As a thunderbolt the energy of the Power Symbol acts like lightning. It works quickly—like a flash—starting to work as soon as you finish saying its name and disappearing immediately once the job is done. You do not have to clear away the energy or symbol once its work is complete. The spiral of the symbol looks a little like a curled whip ready to be used. You can imagine its energy whipping out and then returning to its curled state, when it has finished doing what it has been asked to do, in readiness for the next time it has work to do.

A Command

The Power Symbol is a command that has to be obeyed. Its Japanese name means Imperial Edict or Royal Command. In the past, in Japan and China, a royal command always had to be obeyed otherwise you were sent a white envelope requesting that you give up your life. Besides his Bodhisattva promise to help all human beings reach enlightenment, Vajrapani made two other promises:

1. My command must be obeyed.
2. My command overcomes all evil.

The Power symbol can be used as a command that has to be obeyed. When you use it with other Reiki symbols it makes those symbols royal commands too. The Power symbol has to be obeyed and so therefore it can be used whenever you want an intent or thought obeyed. It can be used for those habits you find hard to overcome.

A friend of mine wanted to give up eating chocolate. She felt she was addicted to it. So whenever she craved chocolate she drew a Power Symbol as tall as herself and stepped into it saying she no longer craved chocolate or wanted to eat it. Within three weeks she had stopped eating chocolate and after 3 months had no desire for it at all. This can also work for cigarette smoking and other cravings. It can be more effective than using a Mental/Emotional symbol because you can't justify your way out of your request; you have to obey the command.

I use the Power Symbol to get dogs and cats to obey. The first time this happened I stopped at an old farmhouse to ask directions and a huge dog came bounding out, barking and growling at me. The owner yelled at the dog to stop. The dog ignored him and kept coming at me. The owner yelled his order to stop again while I mentally drew (very fast) a Power symbol. The dog suddenly stopped, whimpered a little and sat down looking puzzled and just a bit annoyed at not being allowed to frighten me to death. I have also drawn the Power Symbol over cats and told them to go away when they have tried stalking the wild ducks that come to feed on my front lawn. The cats stop, ponder a moment, flick their tails in annoyance and then walk away with the greatest dignity they can muster.

The Power Symbol can be used to turn any affirmation, intent, words or thoughts into Royal Commands that have to be obeyed. However, this does not mean you can make people do things they don't want to do or are not in alignment with their best interest, or are illegal or evil. Vajrapani's second promise 'my command overcomes all evil' prevents this from happening. The Reiki Master symbol, which is used during the 1st Degree and 2nd Degree attunements, also promises that the Healing Energy (Reiki) cannot be used for evil or be sent to anyone with evil (negative) intent. The promise contained in the Reiki Master symbol says that the energy will go back to the person sending the evil intent—not to punish them but to HEAL them of their evil.

To Activate More Energy
2nd Degree Reiki Practitioners can draw the Power Symbol on the palms of their hands before giving a Reiki treatment to themselves or someone else to activate more Reiki energy coming through their hands. Mentally drawing the Power symbol on either the palms or backs of the hands of 1st Degree Reiki Practitioners will also increase the flow of Reiki in their hands.

Use the Power symbol whenever you think of the word activate or when you want to activate something. On a long drive home from a Reiki Retreat I noted that the driver in the car following me had not turned on his headlights and it was getting dark. I began to worry about it and mentioned it to my passengers. Finally I drew a Power Symbol over the image of the car in my rear view mirror and asked the symbol to activate the lights in the car. As soon as I had mentally stopped saying the name of the symbol for the third time the driver turned on his lights. You can also draw the Power Symbol in your rear view mirror when a car follows too closely behind your car and intend they keep a safe driving space between your car and theirs.

I have drawn a large Power Symbol in my living room and asked that it activate someone to do the vacuuming. On a couple of occasions I came home from work to find my son had done it without being asked. Other times I did it myself, and noticed that I did it without it being a bother or hassle.

For Protection

The Power Symbol will protect you, your friends and family, other living beings and also inanimate obejcts such as cars, houses, suitcases, books and so on. It can be mentally drawn between yourself and another person to protect yourself from them. It can be drawn around yourself (with you standing in the middle of the spiral) or you can draw the Power Symbol as a long tunnel in front of you as you walk down a street so you walk through the Power Symbol. Or you can place several Power Symbols within your auric field to protect you.

You can mentally draw Power Symbols around the perimeter of your property (i.e., several on each side of the property) or one big symbol that covers the whole property, or you can place them in the corners of the property. I would suggest you read a book on Feng Shui to understand what activating the energy in the corners of your house or property can mean. Each corner has a meaning and you will activate that meaning as well as protect the property.

The activities of the first room, the one you walk into when you enter your home, provides a major focus in your life. If it is the kitchen, then the focus will be on food. This means that people in the house will put on weight or think about food a lot. My first room is the kitchen and so what I did was to draw the Reiki symbols in the doorway to the kitchen:
1. Draw the Power Symbol from the top of the door to the floor and ask that it protect you from the negative effects of the kitchen—that it protects you from overeating and putting on weight and to ensure you eat healthy balanced meals.
2. Draw the Mental/Emotional Symbol and ask that the thoughts and feelings associated with the kitchen, food and eating are healthy and for your highest benefit.
3. Finally draw the Distance Symbol and ask that it hold the other two Reiki symbols and your requests/intents in the doorway for as long as the doorway exists.

If you want to protect something for a long time or hold the symbols in a particular place, use a Distance Symbol. The Distance Symbol contains within it the ability to fasten or hold as well as the aspect of time. For instance, draw the Power symbol over the whole of your car, say its Japanese name, and state that you want your car protected. Next draw the Distance Symbol over your car and state that the Power Symbol will be held there to protect the car for as long as the car exists.

You can draw the Power Symbol mentally or with your hand, over an envelope before posting mail or on your luggage to protect it and ensure it arrives safely at its destination. Some people draw each of the three Reiki Symbols with a pen, one on top of the other so they look like a scribbled mess, on an envelope to ensure it gets to its destination safely.

Increase/Decrease Vibrations

We are surrounded by a large variety of energy vibrations, many of which work at a lower level than we do and are therefore not compatible with us. For instance the vibrational waves of the light emitted by a TV or computer are slower than our thought-waves, which operate at the speed of sunlight (the light wave our eyes evolved to use). After sitting in front of TV for a while we can feel slow, tired and sluggish due to our brain having slowed down to the speed of the light vibration coming from the TV. The Power Symbol can be used to increase or slow down the vibrations and energies around us.

1. Draw a Power Symbol over the TV or computer screen. Say its Japanese name three times and ask that it raises the light vibration coming from the screen so that it is in harmony with you. Use the Distance Symbol to hold the Power Symbol there for as long as needed.

2. Draw a Power Symbol over each of the electric power points in your house. Say its name three times and ask to be protected from the negative vibration being emitted and to ensure that the vibration of the electricity in the house is beneficial to all living beings in the house. Use the Distance Symbol to hold all the Power Symbols you have done in place for as long as needed.

3. People with metal plates in their heads can sometimes pick up radio waves that cause headaches. Use the Power Symbol to clear the metal plate of vibrations.

4. If you are low on gas, draw a Power Symbol, say its name three times, then ask that 1,000 Power Symbols go into the gas tank to ensure you have enough gas to get you to the next gas station. Make sure you do stop at the next station.

The Power Symbol can be used to raise vibrations of trains, planes and cars. Jet lag, I believe, is reinforced by the slow vibration of the aircraft's engines causing our internal vibrations to slow down too, thereby making us feel sluggish and sleepy. In an aircraft we sit, sometimes for several hours, between huge engines that send out both waves of vibration and sound.

Clearing Blocked Energy

The spiral of the Power Symbol has a circular motion similar to that used for wiping something clear. The Power Symbol can be used to clear blocks on all levels. It can be used on the physical level to clear blocks within the body, in the auric field around the body and in the world around us. It can be used on the mental/emotional level to clear away thoughts and feelings from the past that are preventing us from being who we truly are in the present. It can also be used to clear spiritual blocks.

I often use the Power Symbol to clear hold ups in traffic, to activate green lights and to clear a space in the flow of traffic so I can turn easily and safely onto another road. I also use it to protect myself, the car, and any passengers throughout a journey. I believe that using the Power Symbol while driving puts you into a positive/intuitive frame of mind so that you drive at the correct speed for the traffic and the phasing of lights. You will also have more patience with traffic delays so that they irritate you less. You can mentally send out dozens of tiny Power Symbols to clear your pathway before you start your car.

Many of us have blocks or mental/emotional patterns from our past that cause problems in our present daily lives. These can be cleared away, giving us more energy and making our lives easier and more flowing.

Place your hands on your solar plexus and mentally draw the Distance Symbol, say its name three times, then ask to be connected to the original event that has caused your present problem. Next, mentally draw the Power Symbol, say its name three times and ask that it clears away all the negative thoughts, feelings, emo-

tions, bitterness, and unhappiness that surround this event. (You cannot clear away the event as it is part of history. You can only clear away the reactions that surround it). Next draw the Mental/Emotional symbol and ask that it brings you back into harmony, peace and balance. These two symbols will allow you to look at the positive results of the event rather than dwell on the negative ones.

I have used the Power Symbol to clear problems in the engine of my car and to keep it running until I could get to a garage. I drove for 2 hours with a split in an oil hose. The mechanic couldn't understand how the car had kept going. When I told him about Reiki he just looked at me in disbelief. On another occasion my gearbox jammed while I was driving home late one night. I filled it full of Power Symbols to clear whatever was blocking the gears and to enable me to get home. I continued driving home using only two gears instead of four. The next day I drove to the garage, using all four gears, and once again the mechanic told me he didn't know how I could have driven the car for so long. I shouldn't have been able to change gears because there were several crushed bearings in the gearbox.

Cleansing

The Power Symbol can be used to cleanse a part of your body, your emotions, and a sacred space or atmosphere in a house or business.

1. Mentally draw a Power Symbol, say its name three times, and ask it to send a hundred Power Symbols through every room in your house to cleanse it of all negative thoughts, feelings and energies. This is good to do after an argument, sickness or unhappiness in your home.
2. A Feng Shui cure for cleansing the energies of a home is to boil the skins of 9 oranges and 6 lemons. When the water has cooled drain the water into a bowl that is easy to hold. Then move through the house dipping your fingertips into the bowl regularly and flicking the water from your fingertips around each room. As a 2nd Degree Reiki Practitioner you can physically or mentally draw Power Symbols in the water and also draw them again in the air just before you flick the water off your fingertips. Say the symbol's name each time you flick.
3. Have you ever sat in a chair or climbed into bed and noticed your

mood suddenly changes from being bright and alert to feeling tired or from being good humored to being angry and you can't understand why? The bed and chair are likely to have a lot of tired, angry and negative thoughts stored in them from people who have previously used them. One morning I couldn't find my keys (house and car). After a very frustrating and fruitless search I finally found some spare keys. My employer just laughed when I arrived late to work and said that the two previous people who had used my chair had also lost keys. *Either mentally or physically draw a large Power Symbol over the bed or chair. Draw the symbol the same size as the bed or chair. Say the name of the symbol three times and ask that it clears away all the negative energy held within the bed or chair. If there are lots of people around and you don't want to be seen drawing symbols, mentally draw a Power Symbol, mentally say its name three times and then tell it to send 100 Power Symbols into your chair, sofa or bed to clear away all the negative thoughts stored in it.*

A favorite of mine is to place a Power Symbol on my toothbrush before cleaning my teeth to assist in cleaning my mouth and teeth on all levels—physical, mental/emotional, and spiritual.

Using the Power Symbol as a Filter

The Power Symbol can be used to act as a filter. I have drawn a Power Symbol and a Distance Symbol just under my water faucet. The Power Symbol filters the water as it flows through it and the Distance Symbol holds the Power Symbol in place for as long as needed. I used to draw the Power Symbol over smelly feet during Reiki treatments to filter away the smell. I have since come to the understanding that smelly feet are an indication that all is not right and well in the body. I now ask that the Power Symbol heal the cause of the smell.

Using the Power Symbol on Yourself

A very important aspect of Reiki is being able to use it on yourself. Here are some ideas for using the Power Symbol on yourself:

1. **Negative Thoughts**—when you get those unhappy, angry, or worrying thoughts that run around and around in your mind and won't go away—*draw a Power Symbol and say it's name three times*

and state that it will clear away all those thoughts. You can follow this up with the Dry Bathing Technique, which will also help to disconnect you from negative thoughts.

2. **People who stay in your mind**—sometimes we find ourselves dwelling on a person or people we don't like; people who make us unhappy or angry; people who have hurt us. It often feels like they have hooked into you in some way. *Ask your intuition how many symbols you need to clear away all the hooks this person has in your mind and your auric field. You will usually get a number. Draw the Power Symbol and ask it to send that many Power Symbols into your mind and auric field to clear away all the hooks that attach you to that person.*

3. **Cleansing Body Organs**—you can ask the Power Symbol to cleanse various parts of your body such as your eyes, throat, bronchial tubes, lungs, blood, spleen, lymphatic system, liver, kidneys, and so on. *Close your eyes and ask your intuition how many Power Symbols you need to cleanse your bronchial tubes. When you get a number, draw one Power Symbol and tell it to send the number of Power Symbols you were given into your bronchial tubes to cleanse and refresh them.* You can repeat this for all your other body parts.

4. **Cramp**—*draw a Power Symbol and ask it to send 100 Power Symbols into the muscle that has cramped to massage away the cramp.* If you get a lot of cramps, see a doctor. Cramps can be caused by a number of reasons including a lack of salt in your diet.

5. **Pain in Hands when using a Computer**—it is my belief that a certain amount of Overuse Syndrome (OOS or RSI) is because we spend too long with our hands resting on the electronic keyboard or mouse of a computer. The energy flow of these items is negative and can affect our hands (which need a non-polarized energy or a positive energy). We can clear this pain by *drawing Power Symbols on the fronts and backs of each hand and asking that the energy of our hands is brought back into balance.* You can also draw a Power Symbol on your mouse to protect your hand from the negative energy in the mouse. Don't leave your hand resting on the mouse when you are not using it.

6. **Cell phones**—these can have an effect on our brain because the antenna of the cell phone is usually so close to our heads. After using a cell phone *draw a Power Symbol on the side of your head*

and ask that it clear away all the negative effects caused by the cell phone.

7. **Bumps and Bangs**—when you bump or bang yourself immediately *draw a Power Symbol, say its name three times, and ask that it clears away the trauma of the accident.* I find this helps to reduce bruising and pain. It is useful to do this for all accidents no matter how big or small or how long ago the accident was. It can also be used to clear away the trauma of surgery (which is an injury to the body) regardless of whether the surgery has just taken place or was years ago.

8. **Self Confidence**—if you are in a situation where you feel your self-confidence diminishing you can use the Power Symbol to help regain it. You can either *mentally draw a large Power Symbol just a few inches in front of you, then step into it and ask that it help boost your self-confidence or visit nearby toilets and in the privacy of one of the stalls physically draw a Power Symbol and step into it and ask that it boost your self-confidence and help you cope with the day's events.*

9. **Youthfulness**—actions can contain intents. A handshake can carry the intent of friendship or the intent of agreement without the need to actually speak words. I have adapted the following set of actions to use with Reiki. It has been said that these actions were used by the Yaqui Indians of North Mexico to prevent wrinkles from forming. However I cannot guarantee they work as I did not start doing this technique until I already had wrinkles. I do find they act as a 'pick-me-up' and make me feel refreshed. They are great to use during and after a long flight or journey.

   a. *Draw a Power Symbol on the outer sides of each of your thumbs. Place your thumbs on the bridge of your nose and move them upward and outward with light, even strokes across your forehead to the temples.* The intent of this action is to keep furrows from developing between your eyes.

   b. *Draw the Power Symbol on the palm of each hand and with long firm strokes slide your palms up each cheek to your hairline. Repeat this movement six or seven times using slow, even upward stokes.*

   c. *Draw the Power Symbol on the outside edge of one of your index fingers. Place your index finger, with the thumb fold-*

ed into your palm, above your upper lip and rub back and forth with a vigorous saw-like motion. The spot where the nose and upper lip join, when briskly rubbed, stimulates energy to flow in mild, even bursts. If you are drowsy, rub this point to temporarily revive you. By using the Power Symbol as well you stimulate this point quickly and activate more energy.

d. *Draw the Power Symbol on the outside edge of both of your index fingers. Move your index fingers sideways under your chin using a quick back and forth saw-like motion. Alternatively you can draw the Power Symbol on the backs of your fingers on each hand then hold them one on top of the other and rest your chin on them.* This is said to help firm the underside of your chin and lower jaw.

10. **Pink Happiness**—*Close your eyes and visualize a large Power Symbol, say its name three times and then see the Power Symbol fill with pink light (you can use another color if you wish). Next say the word 'Happiness' three times and see the word going into and filling the spiral of the Power Symbol. Then visualize this Power Symbol filled with pink light and happiness going into the top of your head and traveling down through your body, into every cell, clearing away all blocks and filling you with beautiful pink light, happiness and the energy of the symbol.*

THE MENTAL/EMOTIONAL SYMBOL

The Mental/Emotional Symbol heals in the mental and emotional levels where many of our illnesses or dis-eases begin. This symbol heals more on the level of original cause, releasing negative thoughts and feelings, dissolving and dissipating them and replacing them with positive feelings and attitudes. It is used to heal emotional and mental distress, improve memory and to help you be happy with who you are. It also assists you to recognize opportunities and insights that help you develop your potential and talents.

Origin

The Mental/Emotional Symbol is a version of one of the Sanskrit symbols used in Buddhism. The Mental/Emotional Symbol appears to have evolved from the Gupta (an ancient form of Sanskrit) character/letter for the sound of "ah"; the sound you make when you are feeling completely satisfied. The sound of "ah" has been used in religion for more than 2,500 years.

Sound is associated with the enlightened being (Bodhisattva) known as Avalokitesvara. When Buddhism entered China he was changed from a male Bodhisattva to a female Bodhisattva and became known as Kuan Yin (in Japan she is known as Kwannon) because the Chinese and Japanese saw active energy as masculine and passive energy as feminine. Kuan Yin is known as the Goddess of Compassion and Mercy.

The Japanese name of the Mental/Emotional Symbol, Sei Hei Ki, does not appear to relate to the symbol. Several versions of the words "Sei Hei Ki" can be found in a Japanese/English dictionary but which one is the name of the Mental/Emotional Symbol is not known. Because wood is the Zen esoteric name for the Healing Buddha who represents the healing energy of the universe and because the Mental/Emotional Symbol represents a sound it is my opinion that the dictionary meaning of Reiki's Sei Hei Ki is "Sound together Wood" i.e., Sound with Healing.

The Action of the Symbol

The action of the Mental/Emotional Symbol and its name is very subtle. It works on your inner levels—both mental and emotional. You need to be very self-observant to notice what happens and when it happens when you use this symbol. It can often feel like a deep sigh that is released when you have done something well. If you use a Mental/Emotional Symbol during a treatment, the person receiving it will sometimes emit a deep sigh and then relax.

This symbol is not used as often as the Power Symbol even though it can do just as much and is just as varied. This may be because of the area where this symbol works. The mental/emotional level of any person is private (secret) to that person. You only know what someone is feeling or thinking if they tell you. If they choose not to express their thoughts and feelings we can only guess what they might be and often that guess is wrong. This area is probably the most difficult for us to work in—it can have some powerful blocks. The symbol seems to be able to get past the blocks (the gateways and guardians) that prevent access to this secret area of our lives. The gateways seem to be mental attitudes and the guardians appear to be emotions.

When we first begin using this symbol very little may happen. We are more likely to see something dramatic and exciting using the Power Symbol or Distance Symbol than we do when we use the Mental/Emotional Symbol. This can leave us feeling like the symbol doesn't work. Often the changes that come can be attributed to other things or we just can't believe that a symbol could have made the changes. Some of the blocks we have to healing at the Mental/Emotional level may actually prevent us from wanting to use the symbol.

Using the Mental/Emotional Symbol

Traditionally the symbol has been used for:
1. Mental/Emotional distress/dissatisfaction
2. Depression
3. Relationships
4. Memory
5. Intuition
6. Addictions (though I have found the Power Symbol works quicker)
7. Mental/Emotional Protection

The Mental/Emotional level stands between the physical world and the spiritual world. Therefore this symbol can also be used for those times when our thoughts and feelings touch these two aspects of the world.

In the physical level:
1. Expression of thoughts and feelings through touch and action.
2. Speech—communicating our thoughts and feelings.

In the spritual level:
1. Bringing through intuition clearly.
2. Interaction with spiritual guides and higher self.
3. Recognizing and bringing out true self and innate potentials.

In the mental level:
1. Clarifying inner thoughts and insights.
2. Enhancing memory, study and learning.
3. Acceptance of new ideas and information.
4. Healing memories, old patterns and beliefs.

In the emotional level:
1. Healing feelings and emotions.
2. Understanding feelings so they work for you (i.e., unease means something isn't right; peace means everything is fine, safe, in balance, etc.)
3. Using feelings and emotions productively and positively.

Arguments—*Mentally draw a Mental/Emotional Symbol between yourself and the person you are having a disagreement with, and mentally say its name three times*. Or if you are observing an argument mentally draw the Mental/Emotional Symbol between the two people involved. This will not necessarily mean that the argument will immediately stop, but that it will resolve itself in a way that is best for both people concerned.

Interviews or Meeting People—*Mentally draw a Mental/Emotional Symbol between yourself and the person who is interviewing you, or who you are interviewing, and mentally say its name three times*. If you have difficulty or are uncomfortable when first meeting people, especially on official occasions, then place a Mental/Emotional Symbol between yourself and the people or person you are meeting. You can also send Distance/Absent Healing to the event before it actually occurs.

Remembering—if you need to jog your memory because you have forgotten a name, date, or lost something, *place your hands on your head—one on your forehead, one on the back of your skull. Mentally draw the Mental/Emotional Symbol and ask it to assist you in remembering (whatever you want to remembe i.e., a person's name) within one minute*. State when you want the information because you could find yourself remembering the name or thing at 3 o'clock in the morning. Reiki your head for a short while until you feel relaxed. After using this method a few times you will find just mentally drawing the symbol, saying its name and then asking for the memory to return to your consciousness will be all you need to do.

Studying—*Draw the Mental/Emotional Symbol on the cover of the book you are about to study and say the name of the symbol three times. Hold the book between your hands and Reiki it for a few minutes. Intend that you will understand the contents of the book and will* *remember the contents easily when needed.* Begin your study. This is not a substitute for study but it will help you to assimilate and retain the information you are studying in a better way.

Exams and Tests—*Mentally draw the Mental/Emotional Symbol over the test or exam paper, and say its name three times while you place both hands on the paper.* Reiki the paper for a minute or two with the intent that all the correct answers to the test/exam are brought to your mind easily and quickly when needed during the exam.

Negative Thoughts and Feelings—you can protect yourself from negative feelings such as anger, hate, jealousy, spite, or negative thoughts directed at you by others. *Mentally draw the Mental/Emotional Symbol in front of you, behind you, and on both sides of you, say its name three times and state that they will protect you from negative thoughts and feelings sent to you by other people.* Alternatively, *visualize hundreds of tiny Mental/Emotional Symbols wrapping themselves around you in a giant spiral from just above your head right down to your feet.*

THE MENTAL/EMOTIONAL TECHNIQUE

This technique is most often used on the head. You can do it on your own head or on another person's head. You can also do this technique on other parts of the body, especially if you feel the problem in that part of the body has a mental or emotional cause.

Stand beside the client if they are sitting in a chair, or sit at their head if the client is lying on a massage table. Place your hands on their head as described below.

1. Cup the back of the skull of the receiver with your non-dominant hand.
2. With your dominant hand draw the Mental/Emotional Symbol over the top of the head of the receiver—just above the hair so the receiver can't feel anything. I prefer to draw the symbol physically but it can also be drawn mentally over the top of the receiver's head.
3. Gently press the symbol you have drawn into the top of the head

(crown chakra) and say its name silently three times.

4. In the same way draw the Power Symbol over the top of the head of the receiver.
5. Gently press the symbol you have drawn into the top of the head (crown chakra) and say its name silently three times.
6. Place the hand you drew the symbols with either over the receiver's crown or over the forehead and hold it there for at least 7 minutes or longer. If the client gets restless negotiate for a couple of minutes more. If they settle down, continue doing this technique for a further fifteen to thirty minutes. If they don't settle down, finish the treatment.

The Mental/Emotional Technique is useful during counselling sessions in several seven-minute bursts. You can begin your session with it. Whenever the client gets upset or stuck during the session you can give them another seven-minute treatment. You can also finish your session with a seven minute treatment.

The Mental/Emotional Technique appears to enable a person to let go of hurtful emotions in an easy way—through tears more often, occasionally through anger or laughter. I saw a couple have a huge argument while the husband gave his wife a Mental/Emotional Technique. It just seemed to blow up out of nowhere a few minutes after the treatment started. They were able to say all the things they had bottled up. The husband paced back and forth while his hands remained on his wife's head. He couldn't seem to move them until everything had been said. The anger gradually dissipated during the treatment. Once all the anger had gone the husband was able to release his hands from his wife's head. They were able to discuss their problems quietly and without anger over a cup of tea after the treatment had finished.

THE DISTANCE SYMBOL

Being able to do Distance/Absent Healing is often what prompts people to do 2nd Degree Reiki. The Distance Symbol enables us to send Reiki across distance, space and time to help other people. Like the other symbols, it has more than one function.

2nd Degree Reiki

Origin

The Buddhist Enlightened Being associated with the Distance Symbol is Manjushri; a Bodhisattva of wisdom. He is said to create the bridge from one Buddha to another and he represents both active and passive energy when they work together as one. He is sometimes seen holding a bow and five arrows which are said to represent five syllables. The Distance Symbol is made up of five Kanji characters that overlap.

It is highly probable that the Distance Symbol comes from China. Ancient Taoists of China had a practice of overlapping Chinese characters, in the same way that the Distance Symbol does, to create magical symbols. The Manjushri sutras and texts were translated from Sanskrit into Chinese during the 3rd Century AD.

Action of the Symbol

The Distance Symbol has been described as both an energetic telephone line and a bridge. In other words it is the symbol that makes a connection between people, places, things, events and time. Once the connection is made (by drawing the symbol, saying its name and then saying the name of the person, event, animal, place, time, etc.) the energy of Reiki and the other symbols can be sent across this invisible energy bridge.

The symbol can act as an anchor to hold the other symbols in a particular place or time. It also works to heal the spiritual aspects of the mental/emotional level and can be used like a prayer to send love and comfort, or to connect to spiritual realms, beings and conditions, or to strengthen your connection with God. It also helps change and reform fixed, rigid ideas and beliefs into fluid attitudes that can cope with change.

Your interaction with Reiki at First Degree tends to be passive—place your hands on a body with the intention of healing and the energy flows. You need not make any decisions and you can go through the whole process of a Reiki treatment with little or no thought or planning. In 2nd Degree Reiki your interaction with Reiki requires more active participation from you. You become a co-creator with the Universal Life Force Energy. The symbols do not work until you use them. Reiki does not activate the symbols until you draw them or say them. 2nd Degree requires you to become an active member of a three-way partnership; yourself, Reiki and whoever or whatever is to receive the energy. It is you who decides to whom, what and where the energy is to go. It is Reiki that decides how the energy will create change and healing, and it is the receiver who decides when and if they will accept the energy.

Using the Distance Symbol

In Reiki Treatments

The Distance Symbol can be used in Reiki Self-treatments and during treatments on others. You can use it on its own in areas that need aligning. It is most often used to align the back. This can be done with the receiver/client standing in front of the Reiki Practitioner or while the client is lying on their stomach on a table. Draw small Power Symbols down the spine of the receiver/client to clear away any blocks. Then draw the Distance Symbol down their back. Keep your hand about an inch or two off the body of the receiver/client while drawing the symbols. Start drawing the symbol at the base of the skull and finish at the client's tailbone.

Anchoring

The Distance/Absent Healing symbol can be used to anchor the other two symbols in time and place. When you do this the Distance Symbol should be the last symbol you use. For example when you protect your house you can draw the Power symbol over your house to protect your home on a physical level from unwelcome visitors and intruders, then draw the Mental/Emotional Symbol to protect the occupants of your home from all negative mental, emotional and spiritual vibrations, and finally draw the Distance Symbol to anchor those symbols and their intents in your home for as long as your home exists.

Distance/Absent Healing

The Distance Symbol is used to send Reiki and the Reiki Symbols to anyone at any distance. This is known as Distance Healing or Absent Healing. By using the Distance Symbol Reiki can be sent across a room, to another building, another city or town, to another part of the world, or even to another part of the universe.

The only symbol you need for Distance or Absent Healing is the Distance Symbol but many Reiki people include the other symbols when sending Distance/Absent Healing.

2nd Degree Reiki

You can do Distance/Absent Healing for fifteen minutes, half an hour or more, or for five or ten minutes. How long you spend sending Distance/Absent Healing is your choice and will depend on how much time you can set aside for sending. I recommend that you make Distance/Absent Healing a habit by doing it at the same time each day. Doing it every day for the first 21 days after your 2nd Degree class is said to help you integrate the attunement and symbols, to help you practice and remember your Reiki symbols, and to help you set up a regular habit of sending Reiki to other people. The more you use the Reiki symbols the faster and stronger they work.

You can also send Distance/Absent Healing to yourself. This is a bit like approaching the same problem from a different angle. A Reiki hands-on-treatment sends Reiki through the physical body to heal the problem. Distance/Absent Healing sends Reiki through your thoughts and feelings to heal the problems and works on those first before moving on to the physical body.

Once you have drawn the symbols for your Distance/Absent Healing session you can think of other things, daydream, watch TV, or even have a conversation with someone. Reiki will flow regardless of what you do with your mind or how much or how little you pay attention to it. However, it is recommended that you focus your attention on your Distance/Absent Healing by sending the other Reiki symbols, the five Reiki Principles, intents, affirmations or positive words. Or you can meditate on the energy by letting your mind sort of merge with the flow of Reiki; feel its peace, calm and energy. You can also stay aware of the images, colors and thoughts that come into your mind while you are doing Distance/Absent Healing. These will often let you know what the person you are sending to needs in terms of intents, affirmations or symbols. Sometimes the message you'll receive is simply not to worry. I recommend that, if possible, you do your Distance/Absent Healing sessions in a quiet place where you won't be disturbed.

Distance/Absent Healing is not draining or tiring. Reiki heals and energizes you as it is channelled through you to the person you are sending to.

The Distance Symbol can be used for:

1. Distance/Absent healing to:
   One person or a group of people.

Situations or events.
Time—present, past and future.
Places near and far.
Other living beings—birds, plants, animals, etc.
To people and other beings who have died.
2. Connecting—creating an energetic bridge.
3. Alignment and balance—bringing into Yin/Yang balance.
4. Anchoring.
5. Changing your thought patterns or feelings.
6. Bringing more wisdom to your actions and thoughts.

Because the Distance Symbol can create a bridge across time you can heal situations and events in your past and prepare the way for an event in the future. If you are sending Distance/Absent Healing to the future the energy begins working as soon as you do the Distance/Absent Healing; bringing into place all that is needed for the event to be a success. There will also be Reiki energy waiting for you on the day as though it has been stored in an invisible battery until it is time to be used.

The Receiver

It is the receiver's choice whether or not they accept the Reiki you send to them. They make this choice on a subconscious level. There are some people who do not understand this and so are unsure about receiving Distance/Absent Healing or who may feel that Distance/Absent Healing will intrude on their privacy. If this is the case just explain that Reiki always works for the highest good of the person receiving Reiki not the person sending it. Reiki does not harm; it always heals and moves towards light and goodness.

Distance/Absent Healing cannot be used to manipulate someone into doing something they don't want to do. I had a student who decided her first Distance/Absent Healing project was to get her son to give up smoking because she was worried about its affects on his health. Her intention was good. Three days later she told me she'd stopped sending him Distance/Absent Healing because she had received a strong feeling that she had no right to make a judgment about what was good or bad for him and that giving up smoking had to be his choice not hers.

Permission

I do not actively go seeking permission to send Reiki. I have sent Reiki via Distance/Absent Healing to people who have been victims of war, famine, earthquakes, floods, plane crashes and car accidents without getting permission from each person concerned. *I draw the Distance Symbol over my TV, say its name three times and then ask Reiki to go to the survivors of whatever disaster is being shown at that time. I hold my hands with my palms towards the TV and feel the energy flow out towards the TV.* Very obviously it would be impossible for me to ask each person concerned for permission to send them Reiki.

If I am talking to someone who mentions a problem, either physical or emotional, I will offer to send him/her Reiki. If they say yes I put their name into my Distance/Absent Healing Envelope. If they say no then I change the subject and refuse to support and indulge them in their misery.

If someone asks you not to send Reiki to them you should always agree and honor their choice. In my experience, if someone genuinely wants to get well they will be happy for you to send them Reiki.

It seems to me that the Universal Life Force Energy cannot automatically send healing to someone. It has to be sent through a Reiki Practitioner. However, I have noticed that you will hear about some people's illnesses and problems and you won't hear about others. I work on the idea that if I have been told about someone's problem (physical or emotional), as a Reiki Master it is my job to send him/her Reiki. Here are several ways that I have been asked to send Reiki to someone.

- You get asked to send Distance/Absent Healing by the person concerned.
- You offer to send Reiki to a person and they agree that you can.
- A friend or relative of the person concerned asks you to send to that person.
- You learn about a disaster or accident on TV, in a newspaper or on the radio.
- The person comes to you in a dream and shows you their problem.
- You receive a 'tap on the shoulder' from the universe.

Occasionally I have received what I call a 'tap on the shoulder' from the universe that I consider is a way of being asked to send Reiki to someone. For me the 'tap' comes out of the blue—I suddenly begin thinking of someone I know. Their name stays in my mind. If I try to think of something else I find it difficult, my mind always returns to their name. When this happens I send Reiki to that person. Their name then fades from my attention. I believe this 'tap on the shoulder' is their Higher Self asking my Higher Self to send them Reiki.

On other occasions I have had dreams that I remembered easily the next morning, in which friends have come to me and shown me an injury or told me about an illness or problem they are worried about. When this happens I send them Reiki when I wake up.

Both the dreams and the person's name in my mind, I believe, come because that person has sent out a plea or prayer to the universe or God for help. The Universal Life Force Energy does not work until someone invites it to do so because we have been given "free will" but it can and does, I believe, bring to our attention people and problems that need Reiki.

If you are unsure about sending Distance/Absent Healing without permission, send it to the person's higher self or to their "energy battery" to be stored there until they pray for help or ask for more energy.

Names

Our names are our personal sound symbols and our signatures are one of our image symbols (a photo or painting is another image symbol). The Universal Life Force Energy can recognize us by our name or signature as well as our visual image in a photograph. Therefore a photograph, signature or a name written and spoken can be used to establish who is to receive Distance/Absent Healing.

REIKI DISTANCE/ABSENT HEALING TECHNIQUE

Reiki Distance/Absent Healing is a simple technique.
1. Draw the Distance Symbol and say its name three times.
2. Say the name of the person you are sending Reiki to three times.
3. Place your hands on something that acts as a proxy or witness for the person you have named so Reiki can flow. (It will flow from

your hands across the bridge created by the Distance Symbol).
4. To finish the Distance/Absent Healing take your hands off whatever is acting as proxy or witness.
5. Use the Dry Bathing technique on yourself to ensure you have completely disconnected.

Witness or Proxy

A witness or proxy for Reiki Distance/Absent Healing can be anything. For example it can be a part of your body, a photograph of the person, their name written on a piece of paper, a teddy bear or doll, a pillow, a scarf, a Band-Aid, or a mental picture of the person. A witness or proxy is used to activate Reiki so it will flow from your hands to the person who is to receive Distance/Absent Healing.

Using Your Body

Some Reiki Masters do not recommend using hand positions on the body as a witness for Distance/Absent Healing because sometimes you can feel the pain or symptoms (you don't catch the illness) of the person you are sending Reiki to. I have experienced this occasionally and it has been a little disconcerting, although it does confirm that I have connected with the person receiving Distance/Absent Healing. In my opinion your body acts as a mirror to the person you are sending Reiki to and the pain or symptoms you experience are reflections in that mirror. They can be uncomfortable but are not dangerous or harmful. They will also give you an insight into where the person has a problem and where they need Reiki. Always use the Dry Bathing Technique to disconnect after using yourself as a proxy or witness.

Legs

1. Draw the Distance Symbol and say its name three times.
2. Say the name of the person you are going to send Reiki to three times.
3. Intend that your right knee will represent their head, that your right thigh will represent their front, and that your left thigh will represent their back.
4. Place both hands over your right knee. Hold your hands in this position for 5 minutes (or for a third of the time you have set aside for sending).
5. Slide your hands up your leg to about the middle of your thigh.

Hold your hands in that position for 5 minutes (or second third of the time you have for sending).

6. Move your hands, one at a time, from your right thigh to your left thigh. Hold your hands in this position for 5 minutes (or final third of the time you have for sending).

7. When you finish the Distance/Absent Healing take your hands off your body and do the Dry Bathing Technique to disconnect.

Fingers

You can use the tips of your thumbs and index fingers to act as a witness. Or you can use the three flanges (divisions) on your index fingers. You can use this method for sending when you are busy, in a crowd, walking, sitting on a train or bus, in a car, etc.

1. Say the name of the Distance/Absent Healing symbol three times. (You don't need to draw the symbol for this technique).
2. Say the name of the person you are sending Reiki to three times.
3. Touch the tip of your index finger to the tip of your thumb so they form a circle (you can do this with one hand or both). Mentally intend that the person you are sending Reiki to will receive Reiki for as long as the tips of your thumbs and fingers touch. (Reiki can flow through your fingertips).

Or:

a. Place your thumb on the first flange of your index finger. Intend that the flange represents the four head positions on the person you are sending to. Hold in that position for a few minutes or for however long you want to send Reiki for.

b. Slide your thumb down to the second flange of your index finger. Intend that the flange represents the four front positions on the person you are sending Reiki to. Hold in that position for however long you want to send Reiki.

c. Slide your thumb on the third flange of your index finger. Intend that the flange represents the four back positions on the person you are sending Reiki to. Hold in that position for however long you want to send Reiki for.

d. Part your fingers and thumbs when you want to finish sending Reiki. Do the Dry Bathing Technique.

I know that using this finger technique works. One day while driving to my local library I stopped at some traffic lights near where my son worked in the evenings. He was not happy about where he worked and when I challenged him about his attitude he claimed that everyone who worked there was unhappy. While sitting at the lights I decided to send Reiki to all the people who worked there. I did the finger technique (just using my finger tips). I was able to continue holding my fingers and thumbs together after the lights changed to green and I drove off down the road. They came apart just before reaching the library. I then forgot about it. Late that night my son came home from work, knocked on my bedroom door and told me he'd had the best night at work he'd had since he started working there and he didn't know why. I told him I'd sent Reiki to the place. Jokingly he asked me to send Reiki to get him a pay raise.

I placed my finger and thumb tips together, said the name of the Distance Symbol three times, said my son's name three times, and then said *"if my son deserves a pay raise please ensure he gets one."* Shortly afterwards I fell asleep. The next night my son knocked on my bedroom door and asked if I was awake. He told me he'd been given a pay raise without asking for it. I told him I'd sent Reiki for it. He then asked if I would send some more because he thought the pay raise wasn't enough. Once again I sent Reiki using the finger technique described above and said, *"if my son deserves another pay raise please ensure he gets one."* The following week he received an additional 50 cents per hour because his boss thought he hadn't been paid enough the previous week.

Other Parts of the body

You can place your hands on other parts of your body while sending Reiki. The solar plexus and chest areas are the most often used. Keep your hands in either position for the whole time you are sending Reiki.

Using a Pillow

I use this method of sending when someone is very ill and I want to give them a full Reiki treatment or want to treat a specific part of their body. I personally find a pillow is more comfortable to use as a witness than a doll or teddy bear.

1. Place a pillow sideways on your knee.
2. Draw the Distance Symbol either vertically above the pillow with your hand or mentally.

3. Say the name of the person you are going to send Reiki to three times. Intend that the pillow represents that person.

4. Imagine that the person has their head on the pillow in front of you. Do the four head positions on their imaginary head. You can draw any or all three Reiki symbols and say the Five Reiki Principles in your mind at each hand position during the whole treatment.

5. To move to the body positions, imagine the pillow represents the front of their body. Starting from the top and moving down the pillow, do the four front positions and the knees and feet positions on the pillow.

6. You can either turn the pillow over (to represent the person turning over) or start again at the top of the pillow and say to yourself that the pillow now represents the person's (say their name) back.

7. Starting from the top and moving down the pillow, do the four back positions and the knees and feet positions on the pillow.

8. If you wish, you can finish by doing an aura brush off above the pillow, and/or give the pillow a hug while visualizing giving the person a big hug and wishing them good health, joy, happiness and abundance.

9. Do the Dry Bathing Technique on yourself to disconnect.

Using a Teddy Bear or Doll

1. Place a doll or teddy bear on your lap.

2. Draw the Distance Symbol either mentally or physically in the air. Say its name three times.

3. Say the name of the person you are going to send Reiki to three times. Also say that the doll or teddy bear represents that person.

4. Then do the 12 hand positions as well as the knees and feet on the doll or teddy bear. How much time you have available to do the sending will determine how long you spend in each hand position. If you have a full hour, do five minutes for each hand position. If you have twenty minutes, only spend a minute or two in each position. You can draw any or all three Reiki symbols and say the Five Reiki Principles in your mind at each hand position during the whole treatment.

Using a Photograph

Photos can be used to send Reiki to people, animals, houses, boats, cars, etc. You can use a photo that has one person in it or a group of people.

1. Draw the Distance Symbol over a photo of the person you are going to send Reiki to. Say the name of the symbol three times.
2. Say the name of the person you are going to send Reiki to three times. If you are sending to a group of people, say *"All the people in this photo"* three times.
3. Hold the photograph between your hands and Reiki. Do this for however long you have allocated for the Distance/Absent Healing. If a person has a particular area of the body that is causing a problem you can place your fingertips on the part of their body in the photo that needs healing.

Other Witnesses

A Band-Aid—this is an ideal way to send Reiki for long periods of time while you get on with your daily routine. If you don't have any Band-Aids available you can use pieces of cellophane tape. However, it doesn't stick as long as Band-Aids.

1. Place a Band-Aid over each of your hand chakras (across the center of your palms).
2. Draw the Distance Symbol over each of the Band-Aids and say its name three times.
3. Say the name of the person three times (you can state a specific area of the body if you want as well).
4. State that Reiki is to flow to that person for as long as the Band-Aids are on your hands.

At work one day a colleague showed me an insect bite she had on her arm. It was itchy, swollen and red. The redness and swelling were spreading up her arm. I said I would do Distance/Absent Healing on it. I used cellophane tape on each of my palms and asked that Reiki heal the insect bite on her arm, then continued my work. About an hour later the edges of the cellophane tape were beginning to curl and the swelling and redness had diminished to a small area around the bite. Another hour later I took the cellophane tape off my hands as the edges were curling off my hands and interfering with what I was doing. The swelling had gone but a small area around the bite was still red. I thought it would continue to heal on its own. The next day my colleague asked if I would send some more Reiki because the bite was so itchy. Once again I used cellophane tape to send Reiki to the bite on her arm. Within half an hour the itchiness was gone and a little later you could not see where the bite had been. I let the cellophane tape curl off my hands rather than pull it off.

I have learned that the Band-Aid or cellophane tape will slowly peel away from your hand as the healing takes place. Some peel away quite quickly and others are very slow. Sometimes it takes so long for the Band-Aids to peel away that I have had to renew them for the sake of hygiene. I replace them with clean, fresh Band-Aids and continue sending Reiki. When the healing is completed the Band-Aids will quite naturally come off your hands without you pulling them off.

Like all the other methods described above for Distance/Absent Healing you can use this technique to send Reiki to yourself. This is an excellent method to use if you have a chronic illness and need lots of Reiki. Put the Band-Aids on your hands before going to bed and intend that Reiki goes to the body part that is troubling you for as long as the Band-Aid stays on your hands. This way you can receive Reiki all night long.

A Scarf—this is another way of doing Distance/Absent Healing while you are doing something else. Wrap a scarf around your hand to act as a witness then do the Distance/Absent Healing technique. State that Reiki is to be sent for as long as the scarf remains around your hand.

A Mental Image—sending to the mental image of someone is okay if you are good at visualization. As I am not, I rarely use this method.
1. Draw the Distance Symbol and say its name three times.
2. Say the name of the person you want to connect with three times.
3. Invite the image of the person to cross the bridge created by the Distance Symbol so you can see that person standing in front of you.
4. Hold the palms of your hands outwards towards the image and beam Reiki at the image.

Alternatively, you can place the image of the person you want to send Reiki to between your hands and give them Reiki that way.

There are probably many more ways of doing a Reiki Distance/Absent Healing. The preceding are the few that I am familiar with and use.

DISTANCE/ABSENT HEALING FOR OTHER REASONS

Healing the Past

Choose an event or time in your past that you would like healed. This could be the time of your birth, your first day a school, a car accident, the break-up of a marriage, or when someone embarrassed you at a meeting, which you want healed because since then have you have not had the courage to speak in a public place. If it is not too painful to do, write the event down on a piece of paper. Give the event a title and then write down the things you would like healed. Draw the Distance Symbol over the paper, say its name three times, and then say the title of the event three times. Hold the paper between your hands and let Reiki flow. If it is too painful to write about the event, mentally draw the Distance Symbol, say its name three times and say the name of the event three times. Place your hands on your solar plexus. Mentally draw the Power Symbol, say its name three times and ask that it clears away all the pain, trauma, and negative thoughts and patterns associated with the event. Then mentally draw the Mental/Emotional Symbol, say its name three times, and ask that it brings everything into peace and harmony and allows only the positive lessons to remain. When you feel peaceful and easy about the event take your hands from your solar plexus or piece of paper. Do the Dry Bathing Technique to disconnect from that event.

You can also send Reiki to people in your past to ask for their forgiveness and to forgive them.
1. Mentally draw the Distance Symbol, say its name three times then say the name of the person or people three times. (i.e., All my past sexual partners, or all my teachers and school teachers, or all my past working colleagues, or all my past employers).
2. Place your hands on your solar plexus. Alternatively you can write down the person's name or the name of the group of people (i.e., All my past sexual partners, etc.).
3. Once you feel Reiki flowing ask the person or people you are sending Distance/Absent Healing to forgive you. (Do this even if you do not believe that you need to be forgiven).
4. Draw the Mental/Emotional Symbol and say its name three times.
5. State that you forgive the person or people to whom you are sending Distance/Absent Healing.

6. Draw the Mental/Emotional Symbol and say its name three times.
7. Draw the Power Symbol and say its name three times.
8. Send Distance/Absent Healing until you feel peaceful and calm or you feel you want to stop.

In the Present

There are many reasons for using Distance/Absent Healing in the present. Most people use it to send Reiki to someone who is ill. I have used Distance/Absent Healing to connect me to the right books to read when I first walk into a bookshop or library, and the right food to eat when I walk into a supermarket. I have also sent Distance/Absent Healing to friends and family to find out if they are okay. When the planes crashed into the twin towers of the World Trade Center I knew my son was due to be in New York around that time. I couldn't get in touch with him by cell phone, landline phone or Internet because so many people were using them. I sat quietly and connected with my son using the Distance Symbol. I asked if he was alive and I immediately got the thought and feeling that he was okay. A phrase from a song ran through my mind—*I'm where I always want to be.* Two hours later he rang to say he had flown out of New York back to his home in London (where he loves living) 12 hours before the tragedy.

I have used Distance/Absent Healing to let people know I am running late and please don't worry about me when I am unable to get in touch with them by phone. I am often greeted with, *"I'm glad you're late, because I am too."*

You can also use Distance/Absent Healing to connect with missing animals and ask them to return home. You can send them a mental picture of home and lots of love to help guide them back home.

Healing the Future

I recommend writing down the future event on a piece of paper. Give it a title and then write down all the positive things you want to happen. If, for instance, the event is a trip to another country, then the title could be:

"Traveling to Egypt, during my visit to Egypt and my return home."

You would then list such things as:

Traveling is easy, safe, and comfortable.
My luggage always arrives safely and intact wherever I go.
I am always safe and protected.
I have fun and I meet interesting, likeable people.
People are always honest and helpful wherever I am.
I always get enough rest to be relaxed and enjoy my travels.
I always have plenty of money for the things I do and require.
Transport and accommodations are always safe, reliable, available, clean and comfortable.
I remain healthy throughout my travels.

Try to phrase your list so that everything is written in a positive way. Instead of saying "I don't want to be mugged during my travels," say *"I am always safe and protected."* Once you are satisfied that you have listed everything you can begin your Absent Healing.

1. Draw the Distance Symbol over the paper and say its name three times. Say the title of your event three times.
2. Hold the paper between your hands and let Reiki flow into it.
3. Draw a Power Symbol and ask that it clears all obstacles and blocks from your travels. Draw a second Power Symbol and ask that it protects you throughout your travels.
4. Draw a Mental/Emotional Symbol and ask that the travels are satisfying and enjoyable. Draw another Mental/Emotional Symbol and ask that your relationships with people throughout your travels are in harmony.
5. Hold your hands on the paper for fifteen minutes or more or until you feel a sense of peace and calm.
6. Take your hands off the paper and do the Dry Bathing Technique to disconnect.

I have found that if the Distance/Absent Healing on a future event is not right for you or not in your best interest you will get a message, thought or feeling to say so. The intuitive messages I receive often come during a Reiki self-treatment. You will get a knowingness that the event is not going to happen. You will also not be disappointed that the event doesn't happen because by the time you get the message you have usually changed your mind about the event anyway. For example, you will want to stay at home to attend night classes, or start a new job, or get married or something else instead. This means that you can send to any event in the future and not worry about getting something that is not right for you.

The old adage *"be careful what you wish for because you might get it"* does not apply when using the Reiki Distance/Absent Healing technique for future events. Reiki and the Reiki symbols all act for your highest good and all move towards goodness and wellness so they will ensure you don't get something that is not good for you.

The bigger the event the sooner you should start sending Reiki to it. Reiki does need time to get everything into its right place and right time to ensure a successful event.

A friend once told me that the Reiki symbols didn't work. When I asked her how she had reached that conclusion she told me this story. 'Her husband bought a new car and decided to take her for a drive in it around Lake Taupo (New Zealand's largest lake in the center of the North Island). Off they went and as they drove along she got a very strong urge (tap from the universe) to draw the Reiki symbols over the car. Just as she finished drawing all three symbols and saying their names they drove around a corner and there in the middle of the road was an Electricity Department truck fixing power lines. Her husband swerved and their new car went off the road and down a very steep bank towards the lake. When the car stopped my friend said she just sat there, so annoyed that the symbols hadn't "worked." At that point in the story I just had to ask what had happened to her and her husband. She replied that both of them were fine. 'Her husband scrambled up the hill and spoke to the truck driver. The truck had a large winch on the back of it so they pulled the car up the embankment. If the car hadn't been damaged on the way down the bank it should have been damaged as it was dragged through all the shrubs and bushes on its way back to the road. They only found one scratch, about the size of your little finger, on the panel above the front right wheel. My friend and her husband got into the car and continued their drive around Lake Taupo.'

When my friend finished telling me the story she realized that the symbols had worked. It seemed to me that the symbols hadn't had enough time to work to ensure the road was clear, but they were able to provide protection for my friend, her husband and the car, as well as getting them out of the problem relatively easily.

There are numerous events in the future that you can send Reiki and the Reiki symbols to. Examples are a family funeral, wedding, anniversary, or get-together, a job interview, the birth of a child, education, for future direction, a career, a journey, to meet the right people, to meet your future spouse, a sporting event, or any kind of event. If you have a wish for something to happen in future, or you are planning something for the future you can send Reiki to it using the Distance/Absent Healing technique.

New Year's Resolutions

Instead of making New Year resolutions, which most people don't keep, why not send Distance/Absent Healing? Find a pleasant spot where you won't be disturbed for 15 or more minutes and intend that the New Year will be far better than you expect for yourself, family and friends. You can write down what you wish for the New Year on a piece of paper and send Distance/Absent Healing holding the paper between your hands or you can place your hands on your solar plexus (your center/place of power) and simply send out your thoughts. During the sending quietly allow your mind to merge with the energy and take note of your thoughts and feelings. If you are presented with ideas and thoughts that feel "right," try following them through during the year.

Goals

Write your goal on a piece of paper. Draw the Distance Symbol over the paper and say its name three times to connect with the goal. You can then draw the other two symbols over the paper. Hold the paper between your hands and Reiki it. Do this every day for three weeks. Take note of the thoughts, ideas or feelings you have about the goal. If they feel "right" or they keep coming back into your mind, follow them through. If the goal isn't the right one for you the need for it will dissolve without causing you any distress. Thank Reiki for showing you the goal isn't for you and burn the paper you wrote your goal on.

The Time of Your Death

An important event in your future is your death. I don't know when or where I will die but I do know I will someday. Death is an absolute for everyone. I do know that I want to die as peacefully, quickly and painlessly as possible. And although I do not have tangible proof of what happens next, if there is an afterlife I want to go to the best afterlife there is. So I have sent Distance/Absent Healing to the time of my death to ensure I die peacefully and painlessly in my sleep and to ensure that the place I go to after death is a high realm in paradise. Once again, all you need to do is *write what you want to happen on a piece of paper, draw the Distance Symbol, say the name of the symbol three times, then say "the time of my death" three times. Reiki the event by holding the piece of paper between your hands. Take your hands off the paper when you get a sense of calm.*

Helping the Spirit World

Transitions

Helping the dying to pass over from life to death is an area where Reiki works well. Reiki can be given to the dying as hands-on Reiki treatments or Distance/Absent Healing. It helps them travel through the steps of dying—from the disbelief that they are to die, to anger that they are dying, to acceptance of dying. Reiki brings a person to a point where they can die in peace and with dignity.

A group of Reiki Practitioners were asked to send Reiki to a friend's grandmother, a very strong minded woman who had decided that she was going to die on the following Monday and so had stopped taking all of her medication. She was very swollen with edema (excess fluid in her tissues), couldn't get out of bed, and she wouldn't have any visitors because she was ashamed of how she looked. The group began their Distance/Absent Healing session on the prior Thursday evening asking only that she could cope with the pain she would have to endure without her medication and that she would die peacefully. On the following Monday Grandmother didn't die and she was very angry that God didn't want her. However, a sore had developed on one of her legs and it leaked fluid. It leaked so much fluid they had to use a baby's diaper to catch it. Within a few days Grandmother had lost so much fluid that she was able to get out of bed and she felt comfortable about receiving visitors. She was able to say goodbye to friends and family before dying peacefully in her sleep three weeks later.

After Death

I find that I cannot send Reiki to someone for the first three days following his/her death, but after that period I can send as much as I like. Sending Distance/Absent Healing to friends and family (both loved and unloved) who have died not only helps them with whatever they are doing in the world of death but will also help you with your grieving process. It doesn't matter how long ago someone died, you can still send him/her Reiki.

Earth Bound Spirits

If you become aware of, or are told about, a spirit that is earth bound and is haunting a house or area you can use the Reiki symbols to allow that spirit to move up into the light and complete their transition. Before you begin, protect yourself by using the Power Symbol either by drawing it around you or stepping into one. Then use the Distance/Absent Healing symbol to connect with the Angels and Ascended Masters who guide the souls of the dead and ask them to come and help the spirit to ascend to the light. Beam Reiki from the palms of your hands towards the spirit and visualize a Power Symbol lifting the spirit up towards a large glowing ball of pure light energy. Use the Dry Bathing Technique to disconnect when you have finished. Dealing with an earth bound spirit should not be treated like a battle but as a way of helping and healing the lost spirit.

Haunted Location

Some places have an eerie atmosphere that makes you feel uncomfortable, or gives you the 'creeps'. You can bring this place into balance and harmony by lifting any earth bound spirits that may be in that place up into the light. You can use the Power Symbol to clear away all negative feelings, actions and thoughts that are in that place and then the Mental/Emotional Symbol to bring the place back into harmony and balance. Finally, use the Distance/Absent Healing Symbol to anchor the Power and Mental/Emotional symbols there for eternity so that the place is pleasant for everyone who goes there in the future. Use the Dry Bathing Technique to disconnect when you have finished.

Connecting with Your Higher Self

You can use the Distance/Absent Healing technique to connect to your Higher Self, your Spiritual Guides or Guardian Angels to receive wisdom on how to live your life better. You can also use it to connect to Healing Angels to assist during healing sessions. I have used this technique to connect to cards in a Tarot Card reading to ask what advice the card had for me. All you need to do is draw the Distance Symbol, say its name three times, say the name of the entity that you want to connect with, and then ask your question. Sit quietly with your eyes closed and observe your thoughts and any mental pictures your receive. Use the Dry Bathing Technique to disconnect when you have finished.

USING THE REIKI SYMBOLS TOGETHER

Reiki Programs

Programming is a way of describing a combination of Reiki symbols or a combination of Reiki symbols and intents. The combinations can range from simple to very complex. For example using all three symbols in Distance/Absent Healing is a simple Reiki Program. Placing the symbols with intents on your bed so you have a good night's sleep and to wake up refreshed in the morning is a more complex Reiki Program. These programs can be static—they stay in one place such as your bed, a doorway, a window, or they can be activated by a particular activity or action such as turning on your shower, brushing your teeth or turning on a light switch. Small programs can be set in place to create positive changes in your life—on your broom or vacuum cleaner to clear away all the obstacles preventing you from following your life path, on your toothbrush to ensure you say the right things at the right time in the best way all through the day, or in your inner doorways to refresh and energize you as you pass through them. These small programs can make quite dramatic changes in your daily living. You can use Reiki Programs on all the daily activities that you repeat each day.

Giving the Symbols to Other People

The 2nd Degree Reiki symbols do not work when drawn or visualized by someone who has not received a 2nd Degree Reiki attunement. However non-Reiki people are affected by the Reiki symbols when they have been drawn by a 2nd or 3rd Degree Reiki Practitioner. The Reiki symbols were traditionally kept secret and not shown to anyone who had not done the relevant Reiki Degree. Many Reiki Practitioners still have a reluctance to draw the Reiki symbols or show them to non-Reiki people. This can be overcome in a number of ways.

1. Draw the symbols on a piece of paper then put some glue over them. Fold the paper in half. Put more glue on the paper and fold it in half again then glue again and fold again. Once the glue has dried you can then give it to a non-Reiki person to carry with them. The symbols will work but the person will not be able to see them.
2. You can mentally put the symbols into a crystal, locket, brooch or bracelet before giving them to a non-Reiki person.

Psychic Awareness

You may find that your intuition, which begins developing after your 1st Degree class, increases after your 2nd Degree attunement. You may begin to see auras, make contact with a spiritual guide, receive clairvoyant or clairaudient messages or your gut feelings may become stronger. This is a natural occurrence and a by-product of Reiki. Remember Reiki is safe and does not harm. Mrs. Takata's solution was to request it to stop. She declared it was not the direction she wanted to go. If you don't want to experience increased psychic awareness find some place quiet where you won't be disturbed and draw the Distance Symbol, say its name three times, then ask to be connected with your Higher Self. Affirm or intend that you don't wish to go in the direction of psychic awareness. Place your hands on your solar plexus and Reiki until you feel a sense of peace.

However, if you wish to benefit from your increased psychic awareness I suggest you find out about courses that can teach you how to contact guides, see auras and/or develop clairvoyance so that you can understand and use this skill easily. Remember to use your Reiki symbols to help you. Anytime you want to connect to spiritual guides or higher beings use your Distance Symbol. When you want protection use your Power Symbol. When you want to disconnect use the Dry Bathing Technique. You can also regularly draw all three symbols on your brow to stimulate your third eye and psychic awareness.

To encourage your intuition, put into practice the ideas that come into your mind. For example, if you have a quick vision of your umbrella as you are about to leave home for work, take your umbrella with you. The more you acknowledge your intuition by acting upon the information it gives you the stronger, quicker and more useful it will be.

Psychic Attack—to Disconnect

Some people try to do more than send you thoughts of anger, hate or spite. They deliberately send ill wishes that can cause sickness or bad luck. Or they try to psychically steal information from your mind or to interfere with your opportunities and happiness. To do this they usually have something that hooks into your aura, sometimes it is something that belongs to you and sometimes it is an emotive memory in which both of you were involved. Not only do you need to get rid of the hooks, you also need to send healing and forgiveness to the person who is attacking you.

To disconnect from a psychic attack:

1. *Write the name of the person you believe is psychically attacking you on a piece of paper. Hold the paper in one hand and with the other draw the Distance Symbol, say its name three times and say the name of the person three times.*

2. *When you feel connected ask the person concerned to remove all their hooks from your auric fields. Draw a Power Symbol to ensure your request is a 'royal command' and will be obeyed. Tell the person that as a wonderful child of God they have all the success, happiness and knowledge within themselves; they do not need to access yours.*

3. *Next draw the Mental/Emotional Symbol and ask the person to forgive you. Draw the Power Symbol to ensure this request is a 'royal command'. Draw the Mental Emotional Symbol again and say that you forgive them. Draw the Power Symbol again to ensure this forgiveness is a 'royal command' and that you will truly forgive them.*

4. *Keep your hands on the paper (with the person's name on it) and ask that the cause of the psychic attack is healed. Reiki the paper until you feel peaceful.*

5. *When you have a sense of peace about the problem take your hands off the paper. Burn the paper and use the Dry Bathing Technique to disconnect.*

Psychic Attack—to Prevent Future Attacks

I have found that by setting up a grid of Power Symbols in my auric field they prevent any attempts to psychically attack me. If the attacker is particularly strong I have received a very clear warning and a request for more Power Symbols to prevent the attack. However, I have noted that the grid will also prevent people from doing psychic readings or card readings for you. If you set up this grid and then want to have a card or clairvoyant reading you need to take a moment or two to give permission for the reading.

1. *Mentally draw the Power Symbol and say its name three times.*
2. *Visualize the Power Symbol and ask that it be filled with love.*
3. *Then ask the Power Symbol to duplicate itself ten times.*
4. *Ask that these 10 Power Symbols filled with love be placed within your auric field to protect you from psychic interference, theft or attack.*
5. *Ask that whoever tries to psychically attack you is sent love and healing. You can also ask that they be sent the Light of the Sun and Moon to heal their desire to attack you. (The Light of the Sun and Moon are part of the Usui Reiki Master Symbol, which is placed in your auric field during attunements where they act as protectors and guardians of healing until your 3rd Degree attunement).*
6. *When you feel peaceful disconnect using the Dry Bathing Technique.*

USING REIKI SYMBOLS WITH OTHER MODALITIES

The following are some of the ways I have used the Reiki symbols with other healing modalities. There are many modalities that I haven't used. By looking at the ways I have used the Reiki symbols I hope you will get ideas of how Reiki can enhance the modalities that you use.

With Reflexology

For a number of weeks I had indigestion. I tried Reiki first then followed it up with other methods, including my mother's remedy of a teaspoon of bicarbonate of soda in warm water. Ugh! Nothing would shift it. As the weeks progressed the indigestion got worse and was quite painful. Reiki would ease it a bit but not cure it. While attending a Natural Healing Expo, where I gave people short Reiki treatments, I took time out to have a foot massage. The woman who massaged my feet noticed I had a small corn in the chest reflex area of my left foot. She dug into it and because it didn't hurt we both dismissed it. A few days later I had to take my car into the garage and spent over an hour window-shopping while it was being fixed. As time passed I became acutely aware of the corn on my foot. I was almost limping when I returned to the garage. At home I sat with my hands on my foot, giving it Reiki. After half an hour the pain eased but the corn was still there. I got busy doing other things and slowly the pain returned. I decided the best method of Reiki was to send Distance/Absent Healing to my feet. I used the Band-Aid method so I could send Reiki and do other things at the same time. At the end of the day my foot had improved and much to my surprise so had my indigestion. I replaced the Band-Aid on each hand and continued sending Reiki day and night for three days. The corn and the indigestion gradually disappeared.

I learned that if I couldn't get results from doing Reiki directly on the part of my body that hurt I could send Reiki to the reflexes on my feet. I send to both my feet and to all the reflexes so that everything is covered.

With Bio Etheric Healing

This method of healing works with the fields or bodies of the aura that surround your physical body. It is based on the idea that one of the bodies, the Etheric Body, can heal, but will do nothing unless it is given permission by your conscious self. It can also activate the karmic fields and the soul to help heal the physical body. I was already aware that sometimes using Reiki in the auric fields of the body could shift a block or persistent problem when placing my hands on the body didn't seem to produce any effect.

The first time I contacted this part of me I sat quietly and asked to speak to my Etheric Body. I sat in silence for some time, then decided that using the Distance Symbol (which acts as a bridge) might make the connection stronger and easier. I mentally drew the symbol, said it's name three times, then said "my Etheric Body" three times. I got an answer. In my mind my Etheric Body and I then chatted (I received thoughts that answered my questions).

Several days later I had an all day job sorting papers on a rather low table that meant I spent most of the day with my back slightly bent. My back was aching fiercely by the end of the day. At home I soaked in a hot bath to ease my muscles then gave myself an hour's treatment of Reiki. My back eased a little but not much. I decided to see what my Etheric Body could do for me. I connected with the Distance Symbol and requested my Etheric Body to heal my back and remove the pain. I ended my request with a Power Symbol to show that this was a 'royal command'—that I was really serious about my request. By the time I had finished saying the name of the symbol for the third time the pain began easing and within less than five minutes there was no pain at all. An interesting thing happened. I had not finished the job and expected to complete it the next day. However, someone else finished it off before I arrived at work and I didn't have to do any further bending. Just coincidence? Who knows?

With Orthodox Medicine

Some of the techniques used by orthodox medicine can be harsh on the body; chemotherapy, radiotherapy, surgery and some medications, for instance. I use the Power Symbol to clear away the trauma of an operation and the side effects of medications and anaesthetics.

For an illness I once had, I was given some medicine that caused the lymph glands under my arms and in my groin to swell. I went to the doctor and he gave me antibiotics to deal with the infection that was causing the swelling. The tablets made the swelling go down, but after a month the swelling returned (I was still using the original medicine) so back to the doctor I went and received another dose of antibiotics. I spent a year going back and forth to the doctor about the swelling before it was discovered that it was a side effect of the medicine I was taking. I stopped using the medication but every now and again the swelling would return. Out of desperation one day, I decided to try the Reiki symbols on my glands. I closed my eyes and asked myself how many Power Symbols would be needed to cleanse my lymphatic system and clear away the cause of the swelling. I received a number. Then I mentally drew the Power Symbol and asked it to send that number of symbols into my lymphatic system. Within five minutes the swelling under my arms disappeared. I had to do this several more times. The interval between each swelling lengthened until finally I stopped getting the swellings. I had discovered I could cleanse internal areas of my body with the Power Symbol.

Before, During and After Surgery

Reiki is a wonderful tool to help people who are about to have surgery or who have had surgery. It is recommended that you receive at least three hands-on Reiki treatments or Distance/Absent Healing sessions prior to surgery. Distance/Absent Healing can also be sent to assist someone to cope with pain and trauma while they wait for their surgery.

Distance/Absent Healing can be sent to the surgery itself to ensure every-thing goes well and there are no mistakes or mishaps during the procedure. I have noticed that after sending Distance/Absent Healing you may find the operation gets brought forward or delayed. One Reiki student was recom-mended for surgery on his knee but after receiving Distance/Absent Healing it was postponed, and continued to be postponed, until he didn't need the surgery because his knee had healed.

After surgery the Reiki symbols can be used to clear away the trauma of the operation and both Distance/Absent Healing and hands-on Reiki treat-ments will speed up recovery.

Missing limbs and other body parts due to surgery can have what is known as 'phantom' pain. Medical science has discovered that there are reflexes in the brain for every part of the body. These reflexes continue to send mes-sages to the missing body parts. For instance, the reflex will send a message to a missing hand to clench and when the eye does not send a mes-sage back to the brain that it has seen the hand clench the brain will continue sending messages for the missing hand to clench. This continual message eventually causes pain in the arm and shoulders above the missing limb. Doctors found they could fix this problem by placing the remaining hand in a box of mirrors so that when the person concerned looked into the box they could see two hands (the missing hand being a reflection). They then clenched and unclenched their remaining hand several times. Their eyes saw two hands clenching and unclenching which satisfied the brain that the miss-ing hand had obeyed its instructions and so stopped sending the message to clench. The pain in the surrounding areas and also the 'phantom' pain then disappeared.

I had a hysterectomy several years ago and several months after the oper-ation began to get low back pain; very similar to menstrual pains. After a year or so the pain was quite intense and I was beginning to worry that I might have some kind of side effect to the operation. After seeing a TV pro-gram about missing limbs I wondered if my problem was caused because I had a missing uterus, which each month would normally have gone through a series of contractions (clenching and unclenching). I decided to ask my intuition how many Power Symbols to use to relax my uterus and relieve it of stress and tension. I got a number, which indicated to me that the Power

Symbol would help. I mentally sent the Power Symbols into my uterus (I approached the situation as though my uterus was still there). Within a minute or so all the lower back pain disappeared. I now ask clients if they have any missing body parts. If so, I then treat those missing parts with Power Symbols to release stress and tension.

Hospital beds are places where people lie in pain, sickness, unhappiness and they are also where people die. When you visit anyone in the hospital mentally cleanse their beds of negative thoughts, feelings and energies with Power Symbols. You can also mentally place the Reiki symbols in the bed to speed up recovery and assist with the good health and well being of whoever lies in the bed.

With Mental Illness

The Reiki symbols can be safely used on people who have mental illnesses such as bipolar, depression and schizophrenia. The three 2nd Degree symbols are designed to work in the mental and emotional levels. As long as the changes are not blocked they will work towards making a person more stable both mentally and emotionally.

THE WORK OF 2ND DEGREE REIKI

The aim of 2nd Degree Reiki and the three Reiki symbols is to heal your mental attitudes and emotions, both of which reside within you. Only you will truly know what work needs to be done. Going in and working on this level of you can be difficult. We often have many blocks that allow us to go so far and no further. I believe the three Reiki symbols that are learned at 2nd Degree are designed to help us get past those blocks that guard our vulnerabilities. They can heal these blocks and also what is hidden behind the blocks. However, it takes perseverance.

Include your own name in your daily Distance/Absent Healing sessions, use the symbols in your self-treatments and use them when you treat other people. When you give a treatment to someone else, you will also benefit. The same happens when you use the symbols on someone else, they also have a positive effect on you. Keep using the Reiki symbols. Eventually you will find you have the courage to work directly on some or all of your own issues. Don't be surprised if once you have cleared away the negative effects of one issue that another one surfaces. Our mental/emotional level seems to be built like an onion. Peel one layer away and there is another underneath. Each issue you heal will give you more energy to focus in the now and help you to follow your dreams.

Dreams and Daydreams

Dreams and daydreams come from your mental/emotional level. They are a way for our subconscious mind to communicate with our conscious mind. Often our sleeping conscious mind can understand our dreams so we don't need to remember them. Occasionally we remember dreams because the conscious mind couldn't work out what the problem was or because it is important for our waking conscious mind to deal with the problem or idea that appeared in the dream. 2nd Degree Reiki Practitioners often find themselves remembering more of their dreams.

A friend told me that she'd had several dreams with the same theme of remarrying her ex-husband. She was distressed because she was afraid the dream would come true. She didn't want to marry him again and anyway he was married to someone else. I asked if she had ever thought about remarrying him. She said she had when their marriage had first broken up and everything had been a struggle for her. I suggested that Reiki was asking if she still wanted this wish and as she didn't, she should spend time doing Power Symbols to clear this old wish out of her life.

If you want to explore the world of your dreams you can do the Mental/Emotional technique on your head just before going to sleep and state that you want to remember your dreams in the morning when you wake. Have a pen and pad beside your bed so that you can write down your dreams as soon as you wake up.

Alex Lukeman, in his book ***What Your Dreams can Teach You*** says that we all have a part of us that can interpret dreams, we just have to learn how to get in touch with that part. As a 2nd Degree Reiki Practitioner you can connect to your internal Dream Interpreter by using the Distance Symbol—*draw the Distance Symbol, say its name three times and then say 'My Dream Interpreter' three times. Next, hold the book that you have written your dream in between your hands and ask your Dream Interpreter to interpret the dream for you.* Looking at your dreams can be fun as well as helpful in showing you how and where you can improve your life.

2nd Degree Reiki

CONCLUSION

The 2nd Degree of Reiki is about bringing harmony and peace to our inner world of emotions and mental attitudes. It also helps us to be better at expressing who we really are. The symbols are gifts of protection, compassion and wisdom that allow us to do this work in ways that are fun, nurturing and lasting. It is recommended that you use the symbols on yourself, others and the world around you every day.

For at least the first 21 days after your 2nd Degree Class give yourself the Mental/Emotional Technique and send Distance/Absent Healing to yourself and others.

At some point after doing your 2nd Degree Reiki Class you may feel drawn to explore more. There are now many additional Reiki classes that Reiki Practitioners can attend that add to their Reiki practice and help them explore other ways of using Reiki. When considering whether you want to do other classes about Reiki or other healing modalities I recommend you follow your heart. Attend those classes that interest and excite you because your true path in life will always be interesting and exciting.

One class I found that excited me was a basic Feng Shui class, which taught me to look at how energy flows in my home and environment. It also helped me to understand something about eastern spiritual philosophy and consequently helped me to understand Reiki better.

You should also consider reviewing your 2nd Degree class again and monitoring 2nd Degree classes with other Reiki Masters.

2nd Degree Reiki is a wonderful adventure and the Reiki symbols are friends who assist you in finding out just how interesting and wonder-filled life can be.

RECOMMENDED READING

Books on the chakras. One I particularly liked is by Joy Gardner who was Reiki attuned by Bethal Phaigh, one of the 22 Reiki Masters trained by Mrs Takata.

Gardner, Joy—*Color and Crystals—A Journey Through the Chakras.* Published by The Crossing Press, Freedom, California 95019, USA.

Books about symbols; there are many available. The following one indicates how prevalent the symbol of the spiral is around the world and across all cultures.

Purce, Jill—*The Mystic Spiral.* Published by Arcus Publishing Co., PO Box 228, Sonoma, CA 29476, USA.

A Reiki book that can be helpful at the 2nd Degree Level is:

Kelly, Maureen J.—*Reiki and the Healing Buddha.* Published by Lotus Press, PO Box 325, Twin Lakes, WI 53181, USA, 2000.

Books on other modalities that help you to understand the body and how it works better. One such book is:

Stormer, Chris—*Language of the Feet.* Hodder & Stoughton Educational, 338 Euston Rd., London NW1 3BH, England, 1995.

Looking at your dreams and daydreams can help you to understand yourself and your inner mental/emotional world. Here are some books that I found useful.

Barth, F. Diane—*Day Dreaming.* Viking, Penguin Books, 375 Hudson Street, New York, NY 10014, USA, 1997.

Hatherley, Jennie—*Women's Big Dreams—Resurrecting Intuition,* David Bateman Ltd., 30 Tarndale Gove, Albany, Auckland, New Zealand, 1998.

Lukeman, Alex—*What Your Dreams Can Teach You*. Llewellyn
Publications, St. Paul, Minnesota 55164-0383, USA, 1990.

Cooper, D. Jason—*The Power of Dreaming*. Llewellyn Publications,
St. Paul, Minnesota 55164-0383, USA, 1996.

Chapter Three...

Reiki & Crystals

Your journey will take you to unexpected places,

Full of fascination and delight.

The world of crystals is one such place.

ACKNOWLEDGEMENTS

*T*he memory of the late Diane Kennedy is held gratefully in my heart as a friend and because she gave me my first crystal treatment and introduced me to the idea of using crystals with Reiki. My thanks go to my Mother, Reiki Masters Gloria Warrender, Jenny Laird, and Barbara Pillsbury, and Reiki Practitioners Adriana Simpson, Eleanor Duff, Elaine Mowbray and Jillian McKenzie for their patience and trust in allowing me to experiment with Reiki and Crystal treatments on them. I would also like to thank them for their insights and feedback about the treatments they received.

INTRODUCTION

Using Reiki with Crystals is not a traditional degree/level of Reiki and only a few Reiki Masters teach these two modalities together. To bring the two modalities together so that I could teach them to others has been an amazing journey for me; one that I have enjoyed very much. I found that combining Reiki with crystals creates a powerful method for relaxation and healing.

One of my 3A Reiki students gave me a crystal treatment during which she tentatively tried to add Reiki. I was surprised at how energizing the crystals were and also intrigued about how crystals and Reiki could be used together in a way that was as simple and easy to do as a Reiki treatment. My curiosity sent me on a journey of discovery. I knew a lot about Reiki and very little about crystals, minerals and gemstones. The next step of my journey began when a friend lent me Melody's book *Love is in the Earth—A Kaleidoscope of Crystals* and nature gave me a day of cold and rain; just perfect for staying home and reading. This reference book was overwhelmingly large and I soon discovered I received better results using a pendulum and asking which crystals worked best with Reiki.

I was 'given' several combinations of crystals to use with Reiki; many of them rare and unobtainable. After a visit to all the available crystal outlets in my area I was able to get three sets of stones to work with. I then invited friends and family to come along and receive Reiki and Crystal treatments.

I also experimented on myself by giving myself Reiki and Crystal self-treatments using various combinations of stones before going to bed each night. When I found a good combination I would then try it out on my friends. Although these combinations were good I soon discovered the best layouts were the ones 'given' to me by my pendulum.

I also used Reiki and the crystals together to send Distance/Absent Healing. I discovered what stones not to use and which worked well. They appeared to assist with achieving a better attitude towards every day life and accomplishing the goals we set for ourselves; similar to the Zen philosophy of daily living.

As a Reiki Practitioner I hope you will enjoy working with these two modalities together. I have found their two energies highly compatible. I certainly get a great deal of enjoyment from being able to use them together, and my friends and family have enjoyed receiving the treatments.

WHEN, WHY, AND HOW TO LEARN REIKI WITH CRYSTALS

A practitioner at any level of Reiki can do a Reiki and Crystal treatment. However, I usually teach this class to Second and Third Degree Reiki Practitioners because they can use the Reiki symbols to cleanse, energize and program the crystals. A Reiki and Crystal class tends to appeal to those Reiki Practitioners who are attracted to, and want to work with, or who already work with crystals.

Because there is no need for a Reiki student to receive an initiation/attunement during this class, using Reiki with Crystals can be learned by working through this section page by page without having to attend a class. If you decide to learn how to use Reiki with Crystals from this book I recommend you do so with a friend or several friends so that you can do practice treatments on each other and discuss the methods described here.

CRYSTALS

Choosing Crystals

Many people choose crystals and gemstones that 'feel' good. This feeling may be because the stone sits comfortably in your hand or you are attracted to a particular crystal without knowing why or you like its color and/or shape. I usually use a pendulum to choose my crystals. People who work in crystal shops/outlets are used to their customers employing all sorts of methods to choose their crystals and are tolerant, patient and helpful. You can choose crystals by color or by the quality they impart. Melody's book, *Love is in the Earth—A Kaleidoscope of Crystals*, is an excellent book for describing the metaphysical qualities of crystals. If you can, use your intuition to determine the best crystals to work with.

There appear to be a number of crystals that work especially well with Reiki. Many of them are rare, difficult to find or expensive. By using the Reiki symbols you can program a clear quartz crystal to channel any other type of crystal. This is handy when you need a crystal or mineral that is either unaffordable or unavailable.

The crystals recommended in this book were 'chosen' by dowsing with a pendulum while placing my finger on its name listed in the index of *Love is in the Earth—A Kaleidoscope of Crystals* and at the same time asking "Will this crystal work well with Reiki?"

Crystal Energies

Physics recognizes four basic forces/energies in nature—gravity, electro-magnetism, weak force and strong force. When holding a pendulum over various crystals I discovered that the pendulum would swing in one of four ways that led me to believe that crystals also have four forces or energies. I have named the crystal energies after the directions my pendulum swings—positive, negative, vertical and horizontal. All the crystals recommended in this book, for use with Reiki, have a positive energy.

One of the crystals I was 'given' by my pendulum to use with Reiki is Linnaeite (also spelt Linneite). On inquiring at a specialist crystal/mineral shop I was told that another crystal* was near enough to the same thing. I purchased a piece of rock covered in tiny white and cobalt blue crystals. I tried it out first using Distance/Absent Healing. During the Distance/Absent Healing I felt okay but when I stopped the Distance/Absent Healing I felt queasy and dizzy. I thought I hadn't done the Distance/Absent Healing for long enough. A week or so later I tried again, this time setting up the Distance/Absent Healing to last for three weeks. I sent it to my mother and myself. The morning I stopped the Distance/Absent Healing both my mother (who lived 45 minutes away and didn't know I had stopped sending the healing) and I almost immediately became queasy and dizzy and had to lie down. It took both of us half a day to recover. We discussed what happened over the phone later in the evening when we were both feeling better.

The energy of this particular crystal appeared to be quite different from Reiki and apart from working with the Distance Symbol to enable its energy to be sent as Distance/Absent Healing it did not seem to work with Reiki in any other way. Reiki was not able to overcome the effect of the crystal. We just had to wait until the effect wore off in its own time. When I held my pendulum over the crystal the pendulum swung in the negative direction. The crystal appears to affect the inner ear balance. When distance/absent healing stops, the inner ear returns to normal causing a feeling of motion sickness while it does so. From this experience I cannot recommend using crystals that have a negative energy.

Kyanite and Garnet both have vertical energies and will neutralize the effects of both positive and negative crystals, causing them to also have ver-

---

* I prefer not to give the name because a person I showed this crystal to wanted to use it to make another ill.

tical energies. I have found these two stones useful for neutralizing the negative energy crystal and also electricity. Kyanite and Garnet seem to act as interrupters or neutralizers of energetic forces and can reduce (but not eliminate) the effects of Reiki. I do not recommend using Kyanite or Garnet with Reiki or for healing. I do recommend that Garnet rings, necklaces or bracelets are removed before an initiation/attunement unless they are set in Gold. Gold has a positive effect on Garnet and Kyanite so when they are used in conjunction with Gold they become positive energy and are then compatible with Reiki.

Garnet and Kyanite are useful for placing on your TV or microwave or other electrical appliances. Unfortunately they do not seem to be able to neutralize the negative energies of cell phones.

Hematite has a horizontal energy. When placed with crystals that have vertical or negative energies Hematite will enable them to become positive energies. When used with Reiki the Hematite energy becomes negative and therefore I do not recommend using Hematite with Reiki. If a Reiki Practitioner holds a piece of Hematite in their hand for several minutes or more their hand usually begins to hurt. This is an indication that the energy of Hematite is preventing Reiki from flowing from their hands.

Crystal Vibrations

The vibrations emitted by crystals can be fast or slow. My guess is they have a range of vibrations similar to the range of wavelengths that color has.

If you have a crystal that gives you a headache or a feeling of pressure in your head whenever you are near it, place it inside your pillowcase with a piece of moonstone for a night. The moonstone will allow you to sleep peacefully, yet at the same time seems to provide a connection between yourself and the quartz crystal. It seems to allow your crown and brow chakras to open and relax so your energies and the energy/vibrations of the quartz crystal can come into alignment. Some time in the night, if you are particularly sensitive to energy vibrations, you may feel tiny waves of vibration pass through your body from your crown chakra down to the chakras on the soles of your feet.

It is my opinion that the crown chakra can act as a decoder of vibrations (and the moonstone will help it). If the 'decoder' does not recognize a vibration it will endeavor to protect you from that vibration, hence the headache or feeling of pressure in your head. By deliberately placing the crystal under your pillow you are sending a message to your subconscious that you want the vibration of the crystal decoded and for the crown chakra to recognize the vibration whenever you use the crystals.

Once your 'internal vibrational decoder' has recognized the vibration of the crystal, it will also be recognized by everyone you use the crystal on, as the crystal's vibrational code will be subconsciously passed on by you to your client.

Action of Crystals

Crystals appear to provide a window into other states of consciousness. They allow you to experience their state of consciousness for the period of time they are interacting with you in a treatment, while on your body, while sleeping with them or when their energy is sent to you as Distance/Absent Healing. Once you disconnect from the crystal you will return to your usual frame/state of mind. This effect is most noticeable when you receive crystal healing via the Distance/Absent Healing technique. The various crystals show you the state of mind you need to have to improve your attitude towards work, relationships, health, time, money, problem solving, change and the unexpected happenings of life. Most often this state of mind is one of serenity, confidence, cheerfulness and non-judgment. After being shown this state of mind by the crystals you need to practice trying to achieve it yourself without their aid. Once you can, then endeavour to hold that state of mind for longer periods of time until it becomes a way of life.

CRYSTALS RECOMMENDED FOR USE WITH REIKI

The following is a list of crystals I recommend using with Reiki. These crystals were initially 'chosen' using a pendulum. Subsequently I have used them in treatments in conjunction with Reiki and done comparison treatments with other crystals that were not 'chosen' and I have found the crystals in this list to be the most effective.

I also used a pendulum to determine where a crystal is to be placed on the body (this is shown beside the name of the crystal). However, after experimenting with the crystals I discovered that most of them can be used on any chakra but seem to be more effective when used on the area 'chosen' by the pendulum.

The most common way of using crystals is to place them on the chakra that corresponds to the color of the crystal i.e., purple crystals on the brow, blue crystals on the throat and so on. When determining where to place a crystal I found the pendulum preferred the metaphysical quality of the crystal rather than its color. The color of a crystal did not appear to be important in regard to the chakras.

Gemstones come in family groups. For instance quartz, amethyst, rutilated quartz, rose quartz, smoky quartz all belong to the quartz family. It appears that the feldspar, chalcedony, beryl and quartz crystal families of gemstones are the more effective gemstones to use with Reiki.

AMETHYST—Right hand (use opposite Caledonite or Clear Quartz)

The amethyst encourages flexibility in decision-making and assists in the assimilation of new ideas. It activates the energy to enable re-alignment of all the levels: physical, mental, emotional and spiritual. It has a calming effect upon the nervous system. An amethyst will help to unlock subconscious blocks that are preventing disease from being healed. It also helps to heal phobias and addictions. It will attune to healing forces such as Reiki so it works well with a number of healing modalities. The Romans made wine glasses from amethyst because they believed it protected you from drunkenness.

OTHER USES: Place an Amethyst cluster in your treatment room to broadcast energy to yourself and your clients. Hold your hands slightly above the cluster then draw the Power Symbol over each palm before giving a treatment to activate more energy in your palms and to open your palm chakras.

AQUAMARINE—Throat Chakra

This crystal is a variety of beryl and ranges from light blue to green. If possible get a stone that is mostly green in coloring. Aquamarine enhances your ability for rapid intellectual response and your reasoning processes.

It encourages your innate ability, in your time/place level, to always be prepared. This crystal will activate and cleanse the throat chakra and provide access to stored information concerning the perfection of the body. It promotes emotional and intellectual stability. It can enhance your connection with the higher self and help you to become more spiritually aware.

OTHER USES: You can use this crystal to refresh the air around you. Hold the aquamarine in your hand and intend that the essence of the aquamarine is in the air all around you. If you are 2nd or 3rd Degree Reiki mentally draw a large Power Symbol and visualize the symbol being filled with the color and essence of this crystal. Then intend that you are surrounded and protected by this Aquamarine Power Symbol.

BLOODSTONE—Feet

This stone is said to access the laws of mysticism. It can provide insight into spiritual truths and will promote admittance into the spiritual realm of ancestors to enable communication with them through dreams and intuition. It will also provide insight into past lives.

OTHER USES: People used to carry this stone to help promote courage. It can be used to massage the spine, using a circular motion and working from the bottom of the spine to the top, across both shoulders and up the back of the neck. It can also be used to massage the spinal reflexes on the feet.

CALDONITE—Left hand (opposite Amethyst or a piece in both hands)

This crystal is used to kick-start psychic power and can enhance intuition. It opens pathways towards the expansion of knowledge. Held in the hands, Caldonite helps you to 'handle' having your intuition and knowledge enhanced because psychic power and intuition are often blocked by fear. The left hand and left side of the body are controlled by the intuitive right side of the brain. The left side and left hand are also associated with the Yin/Feminine/Passive side of the body, mind and spirit, and with Lunar energy.

CARNELIAN—Knees

The Carnelian is a member of the Chalcedony family. It restores a positive attitude to life after a debilitating disease and it helps to dispel apathy, indolence and passivity that often prevent us from being flexible. It is a friendly stone. It encourages friendships and helps daydreamers and those who are absent minded to become more in focus with day-to-day living.

CHRYSANTHEMUM STONE—Solar Plexus Chakra

This stone helps you progress towards spiritual growth while remaining in a state of fresh, fun-loving innocence. It assists with the removal of obstructions from your pathway. It also helps with mental time travel to specific time periods. The Chrysanthemum Stone assists with the alignment of chakras on an etheric level.

OTHER USES: This stone can be held during meditation when your focus is on past lives.

CHRYSOPRASE—CITRON—Throat Chakra

Citron Chrysoprase is light lime green in color and is a member of the Chalcedony family. It opens and activates the throat chakra. It enhances non-judgmental attitudes towards yourself and others and will help you to move away from states of imperfection. Citron Chrysoprase also helps to combine fluency of speech with presence of mind. It enhances the actions that the thyroid and parathyroid glands have on fertility and the reproductive organs.

EPIDIDYMITE—Right Hand (use opposite Serendibite or Orthoclase)

This rare crystal stabilizes the lunar energies within the body. You may need to channel the energy of Epididymite through a quartz crystal. The lunar energy enables you to access your intuition and to acknowledge the blessings your receive from the universe.

GOYAZINE—Heart Chakra

This is a very rare crystal and you may have to channel its energies and qualities through a quartz crystal to be able to use it. Goyazine encourages you to respond to situations in your life in a sensitive and intuitive manner. It supports artistic endeavors and enables you to bring your own unique quality to those endeavors.

GYPSUM—Solar Plexus Chakra

By placing this crystal at the solar plexus chakra (the middle of the chakras) it brings together the four directions of the etheric fields, bringing your time/place level into alignment. It improves flexibility in your nature. It is said it will help you to extend your life-span. It also assists you in materialistic pursuits.

JASPER—RED—*Heart , Solar Plexus, Sacral and Base Chakras*

This stone is another member of the Chalcedony family. It helps to soothe the nerves. Jasper will align the energies of the chakras, your yin/yang balance and the physical, emotional and mental levels. For this reason Red Jasper is ideal to use on the Heart, Solar Plexus, Sacral and Base chakras in the same treatment. It is also said to help with the regulation and balance of minerals in the body.

JET—*Base Chakra*

Jet balances the base chakra and stimulates the awakening of this chakra and the rest of the chakras. It helps to quiet fears. This member of the carbon family, which includes petrified wood, coal and diamonds, works on the inter-dimensional level of the etheric body. It has a lighter, quicker energy than its more dense cousins—petrified wood and coal.

I do not recommend the use of petrified wood with Reiki or in healing. It appears to affect the lower digestive system—making the person involved badly constipated and giving them stomach pains. I have not used coal because it is so dusty and dirty.

LAKE SUPERIOR AGATE—*Brow Chakra*

This is the only agate recommended for use with Reiki. Most agates seem to have a slow vibration. I suspect that their vibration does not work fast enough to have much of an effect during a 36 minute Reiki and Crystal treatment. You are more likely to notice the effects of agates if you wear them for several consecutive days at a time.

The Lake Superior agate heightens your feeling of personal worth, and helps you to explore your mental attitudes, enabling you to discard those attitudes that no longer benefit you. It can enhance your understanding of rites and rituals. It also improves contact with information sources beyond the physical plane of this planet and furthers self-confidence in exploring mythical and mystical realms

LAPIS LAZULI—*Sacral Chakra*

Lapis Lazuli helps you to organize your life and your routine day-to-day activities. It helps to overcome depression by enhancing serenity, self-acceptance and cheerfulness and helps to focus your optimum equilibrium.

Known as a gem of intellect and reason it can open the gateway to inner truth and wisdom and help with their acquisition. It is also considered to be a mental and spiritual cleanser. Lapis Lazuli is an ancient symbol of power and has a connection with the Healing Buddha—from which Reiki derives. One of the Healing Buddha's temples in Japan is known as 'Joruriji', which means Pure Lapis Lazuli Temple.

LAVENITE—Throat Chakra

This crystal stimulates mental powers and helps to align the mental body with the higher mind. It can provide insight into the goals needed to create abundance in your life.

LIMONITE—Sacral Chakra

Limonite helps you develop accurate interpretations of the messages given by your intuition and helps you to get in touch with the infinite powers of the mind.

LINNAEITE or LINNEITE—Right Hand (opposite a Trilobite)

This crystal develops within you an appreciation for the beauty of nature. It brings vitality and common sense to the search for wisdom and spirituality. It encourages practicality in the pursuit of your goals. Linnaeite is said to help reduce weight by ensuring efficient digestion of fats and reduction of fats in your diet. (I tested this by wearing a small bag around my neck for six weeks containing a quartz crystal that channeled the energy of Linnaeite. It activated thoughts on how I felt about my weight and I received ideas on how to reduce my weight. By putting those thoughts and ideas into action I lost some weight).

MESOLITE—Base Chakra

This delicate crystal opens a network of communication structures that enable communication with other worlds, mainly the spiritual world, while ensuring you remain connected and grounded in this reality. It assists in the actualization of the chosen reality. (This crystal is very fragile so place it in a light cardboard box when using it in a treatment. Its energies will work through the box.)

MOONSTONE—Right Hand (use opposite Pyrite)

Moonstone resonates with the lunar energy field within the body, which is affiliated with the emotional level. It enhances your ability to receive what is needed from the Universal Life Force Energy (Reiki) overriding any doubts or blockages you may have to receiving Reiki. This stone also helps to alleviate emotional tension by balancing and soothing your emotions. It enhances positive creativity and self-expression. It brings a calm, flowing, peaceful feeling that helps restore emotional balance in everyday experiences. It also helps you to be more spiritual.

OTHER USES: It brings happiness to the environment where it resides. It will help you to come into alignment with the vibrations of very strong crystals. Place it under your pillow to help you sleep better.

MOSANDRITE—Heart Chakra

This crystal stimulates the gift of prophecy and will supplement any skill you have for divination. In *Love is in the Earth—A Kaleidoscope of Crystals* it says Mosandrite works well with Reiki.

OBSIDIAN—MAHOGANY—Solar Plexus Chakra

This stone is black with streaks of brown in it. Obsidian is volcanic glass, not a crystal. It is used to eliminate energy blocks and add vitality to your life's work.

OBSIDIAN—RED MAHOGANY—Base Chakra

This stone is red with black speckles. This stone is volcanic glass that is produced during volcanic activity. It is a 'grounding' stone, providing a connection from the base of the spine to the heart of the earth. It stimulates vitality and virility. It enhances stability in your physical attributes or qualities and will awaken dormant positive mental and emotional qualities.

PIETERSITE—Sacral Chakra

Pietersite is found in Southern Africa. You can channel the energies of this crystal through a quartz crystal. Pietersite is said to enable access to the akashic records. It stimulates dignified power, loving guidance, and promotes loyalty to self, enabling you to overcome any tendency to put yourself down and helps you put yourself forward when an occasion calls for you to do so.

PURPLE SAPPHIRE—Brow Chakra

This gemstone is also known as a purple beryl. It is usually found at the opposite end of a ruby and is often discarded by the gemstone industry.

However, that does not make this an inexpensive stone. This crystal helps to awaken the third eye chakra and also stimulates the crown chakra. It helps stimulate the intellect and loyalty. A Purple Sapphire encourages the remembrance of dreams. Ultimately it brings a feeling of peace and oneness with the universe.

PYRITE—Left Hand (opposite Moonstone)

Pyrite works on the emotional, spiritual and cosmic levels. It assists and encourages the Universal Life Force Energy (Rciki) to activate healing within the body, helping you towards the ultimate state of physical perfection as well as increasing the amount of Reiki received. It sustains the ideal of flawless health and emotional well-being. It can stimulate the intellect, enhance memory and provide for the recall of relevant information when required.

QUARTZ—CLEAR—All positions

Clear quartz amplifies, focuses and transfers energy. It activates clear think-ing, releases stress and creates harmony. Clear quartz can be used to channel the energies of other crystals, minerals and gemstones you cannot find, or are too expensive, or may be radioactive and therefore too dangerous to use.

ROSASITE—Brow Chakra

Rosasite helps to access memory and retrieve information. It assists you to recognize, accept and act on personal insights that originate in the realm beyond normal human consciousness.

ROSE QUARTZ—Heart Chakra and Brow Chakra (can be used on all chakras)

Rose Quartz helps to reduce pain. It also builds self-confidence and self-acceptance. Although this is an important stone for the Heart Chakra it can also be used on all other chakras. It does not conflict with any other crys-tal and can be used with any combination of other positive crystals.

RUTILATED QUARTZ—Solar Plexus Chakra (can be used on all chakras)

Rutilated Quartz affects both the spiritual and cosmic levels by clearing and healing on these levels. It can bring calm, reason, order and balance and also stimulates the electrical properties of the body. It can help increase clairvoyance while dispelling unwanted interference from both the physical and spiritual worlds.

SERENDIBITE—Left Hand (opposite Epididymite)

Held in the left hand this crystal helps you to handle the activation of your third eye. It also works in your time/place level to help you to be in the 'right place at the right time' as if by accident or magic. Serendibite will help you to use your intuition and to stabilize the solar/lunar energies within the body.

SMOKY QUARTZ—Feet (can be used on all chakras)

When placed on the brow this quartz crystal can induce mental clarity, while at the feet it will help bring you back to the reality of this world. The color of this crystal is created by applying heat to a clear quartz crystal. Use smoky quartz that is light brown in color as this indicates it has not been subjected to heat for too long and therefore hasn't become too dense and slow.

STRENGITE—Throat Chakra

This stone is not recommended for direct use as it is said to have radioactive properties. You can either channel its energies and qualities through a quartz crystal or substitute Variscite, which I was told is a non-radioactive version of Strengite. This stone enhances the power of the 'silver cord' connection between the physical and astral bodies and renews consciousness during every moment, helping you to stay in the present.

TOURMALINATED QUARTZ—Throat Chakra

This crystal activates the throat chakra and promotes the experiences of the self as part of the universal spirit. It allows access to higher levels of intuition and stimulates spiritual development by helping you to logically conclude that the pathway is open and inviting. It is good for dissolving fear within you, increasing mental awareness and enhancing psychic ability.

TRILOBITE— Left hand (opposite Linnaeite) Also used for Distance/Absent Healing

This ancient fossil assists in the development of patience, strength and perseverance. It allows you to maintain the pathway that will produce your desired goal. It enables you to do essential day-to-day activities as well as clear out the unwanted without feeling tired or bored. It helps keep your life in order and your feet on the ground while allowing you to move easily along your pathway step by step.

TRONA—*Heart Chakra*

This is another crystal that is said to contain radioactive minerals and therefore its energies should be channeled through a clear quartz. It will increase your clairaudient abilities, enabling you to listen with your heart.

TURQUOISE—*Sacral Chakra*

This beautiful stone helps you to develop the skill of communicating with your intuition while helping to prevent you from losing touch with the conscious mind. It will bring you in tune with those people on the physical plane as well as the spirit world who can guide you through the unknown, protecting while promoting independent action. It brings forth spiritual clarity and will help you to increase and develop your psychic abilities.

WADEITE—*All Chakras*

This crystal balances the mental faculties and 'mellows' any stress you may be experiencing. It can provide an electrical connection between the ethereal and physical bodies, which means it can transmit messages to the ethereal body to release heartache such as a lost love or unrequited love. Wadeite can be hard to get, so you may need to channel its energies and qualities through a quartz crystal.

WARDITE—*Base Chakra*

This crystal will elevate your self-esteem and feelings of self-worth.

WILLEMITE—*Brow Chakra*

Willemite lends you patience and perseverance. It provides a favorable position for doors to other planes of existence to open for seekers, and ensures the pathway is free of obstructions. (This crystal contains some phosphorus and can induce a 'buzzy' feeling within your third eye (mind's eye) when used on the brow chakra).

Other Recommended Crystals

Friends and even strangers recommended a number of other crystals. The following are the ones I have found useful. Iolite and Orthoclase were recommended to me by a stranger at a Gem Show—a scruffy young man who gave me a nudge with his elbow, said "You have to buy those, they're great healers", then walked away. I discovered that although both Iolite and Orthoclase seem to be only mildly effective when used in a Reiki and Crystal treatment they were extremely effective when used for Distance/Absent Healing. The Malachite was a gift from a friend. Malachite appears to be too dense to work easily in a Reiki and Crystal treatment but it is effective when placed under your pillow at night. This seems to indicate it needs a longer period of time to do its work than it takes to do a treatment.

IOLITE—Distance/Absent Healing (can be held in the Right Hand with Clear Quartz in the Left)

This crystal is also known as Cordierite. It enables change to take place painlessly; the change being towards spiritual growth and enhanced illumination. It can strengthen and align the auric field with the physical body and help to balance positive and negative aspects of your character. It also assists in awakening your inner knowledge and can lead to excellence in your endeavors.

MALACHITE—Put under Your Pillow (use with a clear quartz)

This stone will bring dreams about childhood traumas and difficulties that need to be healed and resolved.

ORTHOCLASE—Distance/Absent Healing (or held in Left Hand opposite Epididymite or Clear Quartz)

This is another member of the Feldspar family. It is a general healer that increases vitality and strength. It allows you to move forward on your life's pathway. This crystal will stimulate tact, finesse, poise and refinement, and induce liveliness. It helps you to be more aware of coincidences and symbols and to understand why they are happening to you.

LOOKING AFTER CRYSTALS

Take time to give your crystals some quality attention. Cleaning and energizing your crystals are well worth the effort.

Cleansing Crystals

Crystals have often journeyed many miles and passed through many hands before reaching you. They absorb and reflect the vibrations, thoughts and feelings of the people who have handled them. For many of these people, working with crystals is simply a way to make a living and they have little concern about how they treat them. Therefore when you receive or purchase a crystal/gem or stone/mineral it is recommended that you cleanse them before using. They should also be cleansed after using them for healing or with Reiki because they can absorb unhappiness and the negative energies of illnesses.

There are many ways of cleansing crystals. Because of my interest in Reiki I experimented with ways of cleansing crystals with this energy. After using them for a treatment I cleanse them with a Power Symbol then leave them in sunshine to continue the cleansing process until the next time I use them. I can use the same crystals in four Reiki and Crystal treatments in a day by cleansing them this way between treatments.

Using Reiki to Cleanse Crystals

At 1st Degree
Hold a crystal or several crystals in your hands and give them Reiki. Send them the thought that they are cleansed and returned to their perfection with the energy coming from your hands.

At 2nd Degree
Physically draw a Power Symbol over a crystal or several crystals. Visualize it going into the stones. Mentally intend that the Power Symbol will clear away all negative thoughts, feelings and energies. Hold the crystals in your hand. Reiki for a minute or so.

A quick cleansing method is to draw a Power Symbol with your tongue on the back of your teeth and then blow the Power Symbol over the crystal(s).

Using Sunshine to Cleanse Crystals

Leave your crystals in the sunshine for at least seven hours. You can put them on a tray and leave in a safe place outside or lay them on a windowsill that catches sunlight most of the day. If the crystals have been on your TV, microwave or computer, leave them in the sunshine for at least two consecutive days.

Using Salt to Cleanse Crystals

Fill a glass container with plain salt (not idodized). Bury your crystals in the salt. Leave them there for at least 48 hours.

Using Water to Cleanse Crystals

Some retailers place sticky price tags on crystals. Remove the label and wash away any stickiness left behind with warm soapy water then rinse by holding under cold running water.

For hygiene reasons and to clear body oils, clean any crystals that clients have held by washing them in warm soapy water. Rinse by holding the crystals under cold running water for several minutes.

Energizing Crystals

Unlike Reiki the crystals are not a limitless source of energy. They do need to be re-energized from time to time. Energizing crystals after you have cleansed them will ensure you enhance the crystals to enable them to work strongly each time you use them. If you are doing several treatments a day then energise them at the end of each day.

Using Reiki to Energize Crystals

You can do these methods on one crystal or as many as you can comfortably hold in your hand. You do not need to draw the symbols over each crystal. One symbol will encompass and energize all the crystals held in your hand. If you are not sure how energized your crystals are, check by holding a pendulum above each one and see how vigorously the pendulum swings.

At 1st Degree

Hold a crystal(s) in your hand and intend that it/they are filled with healing energy. You can also intend that the crystal is filled with love and happiness. Spend a moment saying thank you to your crystals for the work they have done.

At 2nd Degree

Hold a crystal in your hand and physically draw the Power Symbol and then the Mental/Emotional Symbol over the crystals. Mentally intend that the crystal(s) are energized and filled with love, happiness and healing. Hold the crystal(s) for a moment and send gratitude to it/them for the work done for you.

At 3rd Degree

As well as energizing your crystals with the Power and Mental/Emotional Symbols (as described above for 2nd Degree) you can also physically draw the Usui Reiki Master Symbol over them. Mentally intend that it will energize and bless the crystals for the highest good of everyone who comes in contact with them. Hold the crystals in your hand and Reiki for several minutes.

Using Moonlight to Energize Crystals

Put your crystals in either a safe place outside or on a window sill, so that they will be bathed in moonlight when there is a full moon. In ancient times the moon was believed to have great blessing power and encouraged longevity. I believe the crystals enjoy absorbing the energy of the moon. To me they seem to sparkle more the next day.

Using Sea Water to Energize Crystals

If you are going to the beach take your crystals along with you. Find a small, calm pool of sea-water and place your crystals in it for at least an hour and a half. Take care when removing your crystals from the pool. Small sea creatures are often attracted to the crystal energy and may attach themselves to them, which can give you a fright, causing you to drop the crystal and damage it. I recommend that you place your crystals in an open weave bag (I made my bag from curtain netting) before placing them into a pool of sea water. Crystals like to sink into the sand and can get lost, especially small pieces. This is not likely to happen if the crystals are all held together in a bag. If people are on the beach do not walk away from your crystals, they may not be there when you return.

Salted Water

Not everyone gets the opportunity to visit a beach regularly so an alternative method is to put your crystals in a glass bowl filled with salted water. If it is a large bowl use two tablespoons or more of salt (sea salt, plain and iodized salt are all okay to use) and stir into the water. Draw the Reiki Symbols in the water with your spoon while you are stirring. Use about two or three teaspoons of salt if the bowl is small.

Leave the crystals in the salted water for at least twenty-four hours. It is interesting to look at the crystals from time to time and see the tiny bubbles of air forming on the crystals—it seems like they are breathing the oxygen in the water.

PROGRAMMING CRYSTALS WITH REIKI

One of the unique aspects of using crystals with Reiki is that you can place a Reiki program within the crystal(s) to assist them to heal. Putting a Reiki program within your crystals will protect them from being used negatively or from someone else placing their own symbols and intents into your crystals.

While giving me a Reiki and Crystal treatment, using my programmed crystals, a friend tried to direct a Reiki symbol into one of my crystals but she found she couldn't remember how to draw the symbol. She tried this on several crystals and couldn't do any symbols on any of them. When she sent the symbols directly to my body she had no trouble remembering them again.

To Assist Crystals to Heal

At 1st Degree

Hold the crystal(s) in your hands and Reiki. Intend that the crystal will work with Reiki for the good health, wealth and happiness of everyone it connects with physically and mentally.

At 2nd Degree

1. Mentally or physically draw the Distance Symbol over the crystal(s) you are holding. Say the Distance Symbol's name three times. Create the thought (or intent) that you are connected with the crystal and that you will work well together as healers. If you decide you want to give away a crystal that you have programmed to work with you, then clear away the connection by drawing a Power Symbol over the crystal and stating that the connection is dissolved or cleared away.

2. Hold the crystal(s) in your hands and give them Reiki for two or three minutes. Say the name "Reiki" three times and intend that the Reiki energy will work with and assist the crystal(s) in perfect ways for the highest good of everything and everybody the crystal(s) connect with physically and mentally.

3. Mentally or physically draw the Distance Symbol again over the crystal(s). Say the symbol's name three times. Intend that the Distance Symbol will hold the Reiki energy in the crystal(s) for as long as the crystal exists.
4. Physically or mentally draw the Power Symbol over the crystal(s). Say the symbol's name three times. Pat the crystal(s) each time you say the name of the symbol. Intend that the Power Symbol will work with and assist the crystal in perfect ways for the good health, wealth and happiness of everybody it connects with physically and mentally. Hold the crystal(s) in your hands for about half a minute.
5. Mentally or physically draw the Mental/Emotional Symbol over the crystal(s). Say the name of the symbol three times. Pat the crystal(s) each time you say the name of the symbol. Intend that the Mental/Emotional Symbol will work with and assist the crystal in perfect ways for the good health, wealth and happiness of everybody it connects with physically and mentally. Hold the crystal(s) in your hands for about half a minute.
6. Physically or mentally draw the Distance Symbol over the crystal. Say the symbol's name three times. Intend it will hold the Mental/Emotional symbol within the crystal(s) for as long as the crystal exists. Hold the crystal between both hands for about half a minute.

At 3rd Degree
1. Do the program above for 2nd Degree Reiki.
2. Physically or mentally draw the Usui Reiki Master Symbol over the crystal(s). Say the symbol's name three times. Pat the crystal each time you say the name of the symbol. Intend that the Usui Reiki Master Symbol will work with and assist the crystal(s) in perfect ways for the good health, wealth and happiness of everybody it connects with physically and mentally.
3. Mentally draw the Distance Symbol over the crystal(s). Say the symbol's name three times. Intend that the Distance Symbol will hold the Usui Reiki Master Symbol within the crystal(s) for as long as the crystal exists. Hold the crystal(s) between both hands for about half a minute.
4. You can also attune a crystal to any level of Reiki.

Happiness

Other energies can be programmed into crystals such as love and happiness. They can be held within crystals with the Distance Symbol.

1. Hold the crystal(s) in your hand. Say the word "happiness" three times. Pat the crystal(s) each time you say the word. This becomes more powerful if you also feel the emotion of happiness while you are saying the word. Intend that the crystal(s) is filled with happiness to work with and assist the crystal(s) in perfect ways for the good health, wealth and happiness of everybody they connect with physically and mentally.

2. Physically or mentally draw the Distance Symbol over the crystal(s). Say the symbol's name three times. Intend that it will hold the quality of happiness within the crystal(s) for as long as the crystal(s) exists. Hold the crystal(s) between both hands for about half a minute.

Angel Cards

If you are not sure what quality to program into your crystal you can lay out a set of Angel Cards upside down on a table then, holding your crystal in one hand, ask your crystal which Angel it would like to work with. If you like to work intuitively, slowly move your empty hand, palm down, over the Angel Cards until you "feel" or "know" which card to choose. Or you can use a pendulum while holding the crystal and dowse for a card. Once you have chosen a card, program the quality shown on the card into the crystal.

1. Place the crystal on top of the Angel Card and hold together in one hand. Draw the Distance Symbol over the crystal. Say the symbol's name three times. Invite the Angel's energy to connect with the crystal and reside within the crystal. State that the crystal and angel will work together in perfect ways for the good health, wealth and happiness of everybody they connect with physically and mentally.

2. Physically or mentally draw the Distance Symbol over the crystal. Say the symbol's name three times. Intend that the symbol will hold the quality of the Angel within the crystal for as long as the crystal exists. Hold the crystal and Angel Card between both hands for about half a minute or longer and give them Reiki.

Rocks, Trees and Mountains

You can also place Reiki symbols and positive attitudes into large rocks and trees in your garden or neighborhood to help them with the environmental work that they do by using the methods described previously. Some people may feel that large granite rocks do little or nothing. Their density means their actions are slow. Over time they can have a very powerful effect on their surroundings. Very large rocks and trees can act as neighborhood symbols; some have a positive effect and others have a negative impact. You can free up their energies, and therefore the energies of the neighborhood, by giving them Reiki. I believe it is just as important to heal our environment as it is to heal ourselves. Our environment has a powerful impact on each one of us.

I used to live near Mt. Wellington (named after the British soldier whose army won the Battle of Waterloo), which was partially destroyed by a gravel mining company. In Feng Shui this mountain would be called a wounded dragon and believed to be sending out negative energies because it is hurt and unhappy. Because it is named after a soldier I think of this mountain as a wounded soldier and I used to often send Mt. Wellington Reiki so it would be healed and happy. The mining company is expected to move from the site in the near future and there are now laws in place to ensure the company leaves the area "environmentally beautified". I believe Reiki will ensure this beautification takes place, which will have a positive effect on the neighborhood.

To Assist Crystals to Channel other Energies

After being "given" the above list of crystals to use with Reiki by consulting a pendulum, I went to a crystal and gem shop to purchase them. I discovered that many of the "chosen" crystals were very rare, very expensive or radioactive and therefore not useable. I could not understand why I was "given" such crystals if I was not going to be able to find them. I decided to purchase the ones I could get and forget about those I couldn't afford or find.

Several months later I wandered into a crystal shop and overheard someone say that the huge Elestial crystal on display in the center of the shop channeled beautiful energy. I had been aware that some crystals could be used to channel information from the higher self or elsewhere but because I was not interested in "channeling" information I hadn't looked into this aspect of crystals. Suddenly I knew why I just "had to" go into that crystal shop that day. I left with the wonderful knowledge that crystals can channel energy.

All the way home I wondered about how I could get a crystal to channel a specific energy. Most of the channeling done using crystals is erratic, unreliable and not specific. I wanted to connect with the specific crystals recommended for use with Reiki and I also wanted a method that other people could use too. The word "connect" gave me the clue—the Reiki Distance Symbol connects across distance and time like a cosmic telephone, fax or email.

At home, with pen and paper, I worked out a Reiki program to enable quartz crystals to channel the energy of other crystals, minerals and gems so they can be used in a Reiki session. I experimented first by using the program to channel the energy of Lake Superior Agate through a quartz crystal. A rock and mineral dealer had assured me that I would never be able to get a piece of Lake Superior Agate. It can only be found around Lake Superior at the time of its lowest tides, and even then I could probably search all day and still not find a piece.

That night I placed a small quartz crystal, programmed to channel the energy of Lake Superior Agate, under my pillow. I hardly slept a wink all night. My mind kept going over all the attitudes, patterns (the behavior we keep repeating) and beliefs I had that were holding me back and preventing me from expressing my dreams, inner feelings and ideas. I worked through each pattern, attitude or erroneous belief as it came to mind. I explored when I had developed the attitude, pattern or belief, what that belief was doing in my life now, whether it was a good belief or a bad one, and whether I wanted to retain it. When I reached the point of wanting to let the belief go I used a Power Symbol to clear the problem away. It was a very busy night. Although I had very little sleep I got out of bed the next morning feeling refreshed.

That morning I looked at what Melody had to say about Lake Superior Agate in *Love is in the Earth—A Kaleidoscope of Crystals*. Among other things it increases self worth and corrects defective reasoning patterns. This is what I had done during the night. I then decided to program other crystals to channel and also tested them by putting them under my pillow or by sending their energy to me using Distance/Absent Healing. I became satisfied that using a Reiki program to get quartz crystals to channel the energies of rare, expensive or radioactive crystals actually does work.

Reiki makes the process of using a quartz crystal to channel the energies of other crystals quick and simple. You do not need to find a special crystal that has "channeling" abilities, any crystal will do although I do like to obtain the crystal's permission to act as a channel.

1. Hold the crystal you have chosen to act as a channel in your hands and give it Reiki. Mentally ask the crystal if it is willing to act as a channel for the energies and qualities of (name the crystal or mineral you want channeled). If you don't get a "positive" feeling then try another crystal. If you have allowed your intuition to develop you may get a resounding "yes" or "no" in your mind. Or you may prefer to check the answer by holding a pendulum above the crystal as you ask the question.
2. If you have not already done so, program the Reiki symbols into the crystal as explained under *To Assist Crystals to Heal*.
3. Next, place the following intents and symbols into the crystal by holding the crystal in your hand and drawing the symbols over the crystal. Touch the crystal each time you say the name of the symbol. Hold the crystal between both hands as you repeat the intents.

Crystal Channeling Program

a. Draw the Distance Symbol over the crystal. Say the symbol's name three times. Then say three times the following intent: *Connect this crystal to (say the name of the crystal or mineral you want the quartz to channel).*
b. Draw the Power Symbol over the crystal. Say the symbol's name three times. Then say three times the following intent: *Allow this crystal to channel the energies and qualities of (say the name of the crystal or mineral you want channeled) to be used for healing.*
c. Draw the Power Symbol over the crystal again. Say the symbol's name three times. Then say three times the following intent: *Filter*

out any *harmful rays and radiations that may come from (say
the name of the crystal or mineral you want channeled)*. I
included this intent because I was told that a number of crystals
I wanted to use were radioactive.

d. Draw the Mental/Emotional Symbol. Say the symbol's name three
times. Then say three times the following intent: *Ensure that the
qualities and energies of this crystal, the Reiki Symbols programd into this crystal, and the energies and qualities being
channeled from (say the name of the crystal or mineral you want
channeled) all work in harmony for the highest good of everyone this crystal connects with either physically or mentally*.

e. Draw the Power Symbol. Say the symbol's name three times. Then
say three times the following intent: *Activate these intents and symbols whenever this crystal is used for either hands-on or
Distance/Absent Healing*.

f. Draw the Distance Symbol. Say the symbol's name three times. Then
say three times the following intent: *Hold these intents and symbols within this crystal for as long as this crystal exists*.

If at any time you want to take a program out of a crystal, draw a Power
Symbol over the crystal. Say the symbol's name three times. Then form the
thought that all intents and symbols are cleared from the crystal.

PLACEMENT OF CRYSTALS DURING A TREATMENT

Once again I relied on my pendulum to give me an idea of where to put
the crystals on the body and in what combinations for a Reiki and Crystal
Session. I then tried the various crystal combinations on my friends and relatives.

Levels within our Energy Fields

As I worked with Reiki I began to realize that there were more levels
within our energy fields than just physical, mental, emotional and spiritual. I was delighted to have this confirmed when I began working with crystals.
My experience has led me to believe that some of these levels are:

Physical—this is both a level and an energy. This is the level
where we interact with the outside material world and with
other people. It is also the energy we use when we are active.

Reiki & Crystals

Mental/Emotional—this is our psychological or inner world of thoughts and feelings. Our feelings are so closely aligned with our thoughts that together they feel like one level.

Spiritual—this level is where we hold our purpose for living, our beliefs about fate, luck and God. It is also the level where we can connect with fairies, angels, ancestors and spirits.

Cosmic—this level is our connection with the creative force or energy of the universe. It enables us to feel a "oneness" with the universe and it is at this level that we channel Reiki (Universal Life Force Energy). During meditation and sometimes during Reiki treatments you may experience yourself flying through space, seeing stars and planets, the moon or sun. This is an expression of the cosmic level. During Reiki sessions you may feel your hands "disappearing" and melting into the person you are giving Reiki to, as though all boundaries have dissolved—becoming "one" with them. When this occurs you have tapped into the cosmic level.

Time/Place—this level is where we hold our ability to sense time and direction. When this level is out of balance your sense of time will either be late or too early or you have little or no sense of direction. Some may say that this level is the equivalent to the natural "body clock" that is a biological part of all living beings. Being in the right time and right place is often essential for living your life well, for your survival and for achieving your goals.

Inter-Dimensional—this level allows us to contact other dimensions of reality; be in tune with plants and trees, animals, crystals and other elementals who live on earth, and enables us to move into other states of consciousness. Having a "green thumb" will indicate you are inter-dimensionally in balance with plant life. Having difficulty remaining within the reality of this world suggests this level needs balancing.

Dimensions of Balance—there are two levels of balance that I have become aware of since doing Reiki and working with crystals. They are:

1. **Yin/Yang**—the feminine (passive) and masculine (active) aspects of a person.
2. **Lunar/Solar**—the intuitive and rational sides of your mind and body.

The Layouts

The following are a number of crystal layouts that I found beneficial when using crystals with Reiki. They follow the main chakra system.

The Physical/Emotional Layout

ACTION	LAYOUT	CRYSTAL
This set of crystals works with Reiki to bring about healing and balance to the physical and emotional levels and to the solar and lunar energies. It also enhances self-expression.	Brow	Purple Sapphire
	Throat	Aquamarine
	Heart	Rose Quartz
	Solar Plexus	Rutilated Crystal
	Sacral	Lapis Lazuli
	Base	Red Obsidian
	Right Hand	Moonstone
	Left Hand	Pyrite

The Mental/Spiritual Layout

ACTION	LAYOUT	CRYSTAL
This set of crystals works to bring self-confidence and flexibility, increase intuition and stimulates spiritual development.	Brow	Lake Superior Agate
	Throat	Tourmalinated Quartz
	Heart	Mosandrite
	Solar Plexus	Mahogany Obsidian
	Sacral	Turquoise
	Base	Jet
	Right Hand	Amethyst
	Left Hand	Caledonite

The Time/Place Layout

ACTION	LAYOUT	CRYSTAL
The crystals in this set work to increase flexibility, stabilize solar and lunar energies, further intuitive abilities, increase abundance in your life and stimulate the mind. It also balances the body clock and sense of direction.	Brow	Rosasite
	Throat	Lavenite
	Heart	Trona
	Solar Plexus	Gypsum
	Sacral	Limonite
	Base	Wardite
	Right Hand	Epididymite
	Left Hand	Serendibite

The Life Path Layout

ACTION	LAYOUT	CRYSTAL
These crystals bring into awareness your quest in life and support your creative activities, helping you to reach your goals. They enhance your spiritual connection and help you to receive guidance about your quest.	Brow	Willemite
	Throat	Strengite
	Heart	Goyazite
	Solar Plexus	Chrysanthemum Stone
	Sacral	Pietersite
	Base	Mesolite
	Right Hand	Linnacite
	Left Hand	Trilobite

I was often directed to other crystals that would help the healing process. Not all crystals heal. Some work to improve intuition, others assist meditation or will answer questions or take you into different realities. Because Reiki is a natural healing process I have chosen to work with those crystals that heal the body physically, mentally and emotionally or that balance chakras or other energy fields.

The Chalcedony Layout—Chakra Balance

ACTION	LAYOUT	CRYSTAL
This set of crystals balance the chakras, relaxes and soothes. They also balance mentally and emotionally. They can bring out old unhealed family related problems and emotions safely.	Brow	Rose Quartz
	Throat	Citron Chrysoprase
	Heart	Red Jasper
	Solar Plexus	Red Jasper
	Sacral	Red Jasper
	Base	Red Jasper
	Left & Right Hands	Chalcedony
	Knees (both)	Carnelian
	Between the Ankles	Bloodstone

The Quartz Layout—Mental/Emotional Balance

For this layout it is recommended that you use small quartz crystals or clusters for the brow and throat and use larger crystals (about the size you can hold comfortably in your hand) for the other positions.

ACTION	LAYOUT	CRYSTAL
This arrangement of	Brow	Clear Quartz
quartz crystals amplifies	Throat	Tourmalinated Quartz
and works in harmony	Heart	Rose Quartz
with Reiki where needed	Solar Plexus	Rutilated Quartz
and ensures the receiver	Sacral	Clear Quartz
is refreshed, energized,	Base	Clear Quartz
grounded and emotional-	Right Hand	Amethyst
ly balanced.	Left Hand	Clear Quartz

You can change the crystals around and use them in different positions and different combinations. Follow your intuition when you are working with the crystals. You can also use crystals based on the colors of the chakras (which are described in most books about crystals) with a Reiki treatment.

The action of any crystal can be enhanced by placing four small quartz crystals around it. Place a quartz in each of the four directions (east, south, west, north) around the crystal you want enhanced with their points directed at the center stone.

REIKI AND CRYSTAL TREATMENTS

Number of Treatments

It is recommended your client receives a minimum of four Reiki and Crystal treatments. You can use the same set of crystals for all four treatments or you can use a different set of crystals for each of the treatments you give yourself or your client. If you intend to give yourself or a client more than four Reiki and Crystal treatments you need to use a different set of crystals for the extra treatments.

It seems that by the 4th treatment with the same crystals the body is brought into alignment with the crystals and there is nothing more for the crystals to do. A month or so later you will find that you can use those same crystals again because their effect has been diluted by the day-to-day ups and downs of life.

Length of Treatment

Crystals will almost cut the time of a Reiki treatment in half. A Reiki and crystal treatment lasts 35 minutes. I personally do the treatment for 36 minutes. I discovered that if you do the treatment in less than 35 minutes i.e., 34 or less, the person receiving the treatment will feel groggy and a little disoriented when they get off the massage table. If you take a minute more than 35 minutes to do a treatment most people will get off the table alert and bright. However, I have noticed that if a client chats at the beginning of the treatment the time of the treatment will be longer—basically it will take 35 minutes from the time they stop talking.

Using a Table

Because you are going to be placing stones and crystals on the receiver/client's body they will need to lie down. The best place is on a massage table. Make sure they are warm and comfortable:
1. they do not need to remove any clothes.
2. cover them with a light blanket if it is cold.

The treatment is usually done with the receiver/client lying on their back, so check to see if they need support under their knees. Some people may prefer to lie on their stomach. If this is the case, ensure they are comfortable—that their spine is straight and their arms are in a comfortable position. I prefer to place the crystal layout down the front of the client. I found the crystals seem to be more effective when they are placed on the front of the body rather than on a person's back.

Where to Place the Crystals

Regardless of whether the receiver/client is lying on their back or their stomach, place the crystals on the chakra points down the center of their body. Crystals are placed on the brow, throat, solar plexus, sacral, and base chakras and in each hand. You can also place them on the knees, shoulders and at the feet (on the table between the ankles). There is no need to place a crystal at the crown chakra because you will be doing Reiki on the four head positions and that seems to compensate for having no crystal at the crown chakra.

Once the receiver/client is comfortable on the table start placing the crystals on their body from the feet upwards so that the last crystal put into place is on their brow.

When you take the crystals off the client at the end of the treatment start at the brow and end at the feet. After you take the crystals off the receiver/client, hold all of them in your hand and draw a Power Symbol over them; say the symbol's name three times; then intend that the crystals are cleansed. Hold the crystals between both hands and Reiki them for a moment or two.

Hand Positions for a Reiki and Crystal Treatment

I have found you only need to give Reiki to the head, throat, upper chest and feet during a Reiki and crystal treatment. By placing a chair at each end of the massage table you can be seated during the treatment. These hand positions are only a guide. You may want to use different ones.

Divide the length of the treatment (36 minutes) by the number of hand positions (6 hand positions) to give you the number of minutes to spend at each hand position (i.e., 6 minutes). The hand positions I use are:
1. Hands over eyes.
2. Hands on temples.
3. Hands under head (press your hands into the pillow and slide your hands under the head instead of rolling the head to get your hands into place. Be careful not to knock the crystal off the brow chakra).
4. Hands over throat.
5. Hands over the upper chest.
6. Hands on the feet (use a position that is comfortable for your hands).

At 2nd and 3rd Degree Levels

Reiki Practitioners who have done the 2nd and 3rd Degrees of Reiki can use the Reiki symbols, the mental/emotional technique, and the Power Symbol to cleanse body organs. The Happiness Power Symbol is a lovely way to finish a treatment. I also include the following program:

Immune System Pick-Me-Up—close your eyes and ask how many Power symbols your receiver/client needs to assist their immune system to clear their body of infection, parasites, harmful bacteria and viruses. When you receive a number from your intuition then: *Mentally draw a Power Symbol and say its name three times. Then say that you want (state the number you were given) Power Symbols to go into their immune system to assist it with ridding their body of infection, harmful bacteria, parasites and viruses (or you can state a specific infection i.e., cold, candida, etc.)*

After a Reiki and Crystal treatment do the Dry Bathing Technique on yourself to disconnect then give your client a glass of water. It is recommended that you drink some water as well after giving a Reiki and crystal treatment.

Self-Treatments

It is easy to combine a Reiki self-treatment with crystals. Here are three methods that I have used. You may discover other ways of giving yourself a Reiki and crystal self-treatment. The Power Symbol Cleanse, the Immune System Pick-Me-Up and the Happiness Power Symbol can also be used during your own self-treatments. Using them will not only promote healing but will also help you practice using your intuition while learning to trust the answers you are given.

1. Make a circle on the floor with some large quartz crystals. Have the points of the crystals facing into the circle. Position the crystals so they are directly opposite a crystal on the other side of the circle. Have one pair of crystals aligned north/south and another pair aligned east/west. Ensure the circle is big enough for you to either sit in or lie in. Place yourself inside the circle (either lying down or sitting). Do the hand positions for a Reiki Self-treatment. Alternatively sit in the circle and place your hands on your thighs (to give yourself Reiki) and meditate.

2. Lie on your bed and place the crystals you have chosen (or use one of the layouts in this book) on your chakras. Place the crystals at your feet first then move up your body placing crystals on your knees, base, sacral, solar plexus, heart, throat and brow chakras and finally hold a crystal in each hand. Next mentally draw the Distance Symbol and ask that Reiki be sent to each of the Reiki

hand positions on your body for as long as the crystals are on your body. Then place your hands (holding crystals) against your sides (you will feel them warm and send Reiki into your body). Close your eyes and relax. This treatment will take about 36 minutes. When you feel you want to open your eyes and you feel awake and alert, you can end the treatment. I like to do this self-treatment before going to sleep at night. Although I often doze during this treatment it does not prevent me from having a good night's sleep. In fact I believe it helps me sleep better.

REIKI AND CRYSTAL DISTANCE/ABSENT HEALING

Combining crystals with Reiki Distance/Absent Healing is very easy and most crystals can be used. They can be used one at a time or several together. You can try various combinations of crystals to see which you prefer. I suggest you experiment by placing your own name in your Distance/Absent Healing envelope or book, keep a record of which crystals you use and monitor how you feel each day. Begin by using one crystal by itself and then later try using it with several other crystals at the same time.

One combination I personally tried and could not recommend, but which was recommended in a book about crystals, was Moonstone and Rose Quartz. I found that I was kind of day-dreamy and "out of it", lacking attention or interest in what I was doing. I felt this could possibly be an unsafe combination to use for people who might be driving or working with dangerous tools, etc. This combination seems to work better when placed under your pillow, ensuring a relaxed and pleasant night's sleep.

Another crystal I do not like using for Distance/Absent Healing is Amethyst. At the end of a day using Amethyst I felt drained of energy, almost as if I had been giving energy away to everyone I met. Yet I had some quite unexpected meetings with old friends and interacted with more people during the day than I normally would. The Amethyst is a very "giving" crystal. It works really well as a cluster in your healing/treatment room where it can send energy to yourself and everyone you work with during the day.

Reiki & Crystals

The Crystal Distance/Absent Healing Technique

Sometimes you do not have a lot of time to send Reiki Distance/Absent Healing to people who have requested it. This is when I find sending Distance/Absent Healing using crystals very handy. The Distance symbol assists with the connection between the crystals and the person or people receiving the healing but the energy that crosses the energetic bridge formed by the Distance symbol is the energy flowing from the crystals and the symbols you have programd into them. Because you have programd your crystals with the Reiki symbols, the energy flowing from the crystals is safe and will work for the benefit of the person or people receiving the energy.

Like Reiki, Crystal Distance/Absent Healing can be sent to one person or to many people. You can use a photograph or write a name or names on a piece paper to act as a surrogate for the person(s) requiring the healing.

1. Write the name of a person (or several people) on a piece of paper. Alternatively, obtain a photo of the person or people. You can also write the names of each person on individual pieces of paper and then put all the pieces into an envelope; or you can use a book of photos.
2. Select a crystal or a group of crystals. You can choose them because of their qualities or just because you intuitively feel they are right for the healing.
3. Place the crystals on the paper, envelope, photo or book of photos.
4. Hold the crystals on top of the paper/photo in one hand. With the other hand draw the Distance Symbol over the crystals. Say the name of the symbol three times then say: *"Send healing energy to (name of the person) for as long as these crystals sit on this paper/photo,"* three times. If you have listed names on a sheet of paper or put them into an envelope then say three times: *"Send healing energy to all the people whose names are listed on this paper/in this envelope for as long as these crystals sit on this paper/envelope."* Or, if you use a book of photos, say: *"Send healing energy to all the people who are in these photos for as long as these crystals sit on this book of photos."*

5. Hold your hands over the crystals and paper/envelope/photo/book of photos for as long as you want to. While you are doing this you are also sending Reiki from your hands as well as the energy of the crystals and the Reiki programd into the crystals.

6. Put your paper, envelope, photo or book of photos with the crystals still on top in a place where they won't be disturbed. If you place them in either sunlight or moonlight you can state that the healing energies of sunlight or moonlight or both will also be sent with the Crystal Distance/Absent Healing.

7. You can now leave the paper, envelope, photo or book of photos and crystals there for as long as you like. You can change the crystals daily, weekly or monthly. I have sent Distance/Absent healing for six consecutive weeks using the same crystals. After that I could feel their energy get weaker. The crystals do not have infinite energy so they have to rest, be cleansed and re-energized from time to time. Each time you change the crystals you need to do the Crystal Distance/Absent Healing technique (as described above) again.

Following are some of the crystals that I have used for Distance/Absent Healing.

Clear Quartz Cluster

This is a cluster of small crystals that can be held comfortably in the hand. Although I have used clusters on their own for Distance/Absent Healing I find it more effective to use them in conjunction with another type of crystal. On its own quartz crystal seems to have a kind of unfocused energy. Although I felt I had plenty of energy when I was receiving a clear quartz Distance/Absent Healing, I tended to waste it—not finishing anything and often spending time just wondering what to do for the day. When using quartz with another crystal or stone it is the other crystal or stone and not the quartz that appears to provide the focus for the energy.

Orthoclase and Clear Quartz Cluster

This combination appears to send a flow of energy that lets you move through your day in an easy constant way (your day doesn't feel as if it has been broken up into bits and pieces or sections). The mind is alert and nothing seems to be too much trouble. You are able to see the humor in things that happen during the day and are less likely to be on the defensive when dealing with people. You find yourself drawing like-minded people into your life. At no time do you feel rushed, nothing is a hassle, but everything seems to get done that needs to get done.

Trilobite

I just love this little fellow. I use this ancient fossil on days when I want to tidy up my house, filing cabinet, long forgotten cupboards or clean out and let go of old emotional rubbish I may have been hanging on to. The energy it provides has a "quicker, stronger" feel to it than the combination of the Orthoclase and Clear Quartz. It does not need the extra energy of the Clear Quartz so I use the Trilobite on its own for Distance/Absent Healing. If you have not set yourself some cleaning tasks for the day you will often find yourself unexpectedly cleaning forgotten corners or cupboards.

I experimented with the Trilobite by sending its energy by Distance/Absent Healing to my mother, friends and myself several times. The results were always the same—even though I never told my mother which stone or crystal I was using, after the first couple of occasions my mother always knew when I was using the Trilobite. On one occasion she rang to say she knew I was sending Distance/Absent Healing with the Trilobite because she had gotten half-way through her vacuuming that morning then stopped to clear and tidy her dresser drawers and completely forgot about vacuum cleaning. It seems that dusty floors were of no concern to the Trilobite.

A friend who often said Distance/Absent Healing didn't work on her allowed me to send her a Crystal Distance/Absent Healing. I used the Trilobite for a week (she didn't know which crystal I used). A day after the Distance/Absent Healing began, as she was about to go to bed for the night, she suddenly decided to clean and tidy her kitchen cupboards. Two hours later she went to bed pleased her cupboards were so tidy, surprised that she wasn't exhausted and delighted that she had finished what she had started.

The Trilobite appears to have been a fussy little fellow who liked his environment to be very tidy. It seems to have had a very "Zen" approach to daily living. You are able to get through a great deal of work without feeling tired or bored, and you get a lot of satisfaction from doing the many jobs you have often put aside through lack of interest or because you thought they were too hard. After using the Trilobite for Distance/Absent Healing I am not surprised that the Trilobite was the most successful living creature during the Cambrian period nearly 500 million years ago.

Iolite and Clear Quartz Cluster

This combination appears to help you undertake bigger tasks such as shifting furniture around your house or doing the springtime clearing in your garden. It will also help with mental tasks such as writing letters, reports and making plans. All the crystals I recommend here for Distance/Absent Healing enable you to do your work well and to feel satisfied with what you have done. I have found that the work done on the days when using Iolite and Clear Quartz often brings praise from other people—sometimes because the work is big enough to be seen by others but more often because somehow you bring a creative flair to what you do.

Rose Quartz and Clear Quartz Cluster

This combination has a peaceful energy. Although it allows you to stay focused on what you are doing you won't feel any task is very urgent and you will tend to get through the day happily, easily and with a "she'll be right, mate" attitude. These crystals are for the days you don't have any particular tasks to perform—great for holidays when you just want to relax and rest. You may find you attract people to you or you have small moments of good luck—finding coins or receiving flowers, etc. At night this combination helps you relax and sleep peacefully.

Chrysanthemum Stone and Clear Quartz Cluster

I found this combination is best used at night. It has a gentle energy. It feels peaceful and relaxing. I find it helps to provide a good night's sleep. Dreams are peaceful and you awake feeling refreshed.

Crystal Layouts

Any of the crystal layouts that appear in this book can be used for Distance/Absent Healing. Or you may prefer to select your own. Select the crystals for what they can do rather than their colors. If you have someone who has had an operation on their throat, for instance, you can use several crystals that heal the throat such as Aquamarine, Citron Chrysoprase and Tourmalinated Quartz with a Rose Quartz to reduce pain and a clear quartz for general overall healing.

If you are not sure what a crystal or a group of crystals will do, send their energy as Distance/Absent Healing to yourself and observe what happens to you.

CRYSTALS UNDER YOUR PILLOW

You can place any of the crystals under your pillow and sleep on them. This is another good way of getting to know your crystals. Place the crystal inside your pillow slip so it doesn't get lost. Here are some crystals I have used under my pillow.

Bloodstone

This stone allows you to dream of your past, not just this life but previous lives as well. I dream of Egypt, where I believe I lived several past lives, when I have this stone under my pillow. It will also bring your attention to family patterns which may not be beneficial to you—such as poverty or marriage patterns you have inherited from an ancestor that are creating blocks or upsets in your life. These patterns can often be passed down through families for generations. As you are falling off to sleep or when you wake in the morning, you may find your mind drifting to a family member or members who have a similar pattern as you. It may cause some tears to flow if the pattern is particularly difficult. If this should happen then:

Close your eyes, place your hands on your solar plexus, and ask which ancestor this pattern originally came from. When you get a name or image mentally draw the Distance Symbol, say its name three times, then say your ancestor's name three times. If you don't know their actual name you can say "Great Grandfather on my mother's side" or "My Paternal Grandmother", etc. Then mentally draw the Distance Symbol again, say its name three times and say "Myself and all my family in all generations who have inherited this pattern" three times. Next mentally draw a Power Symbol, say its name three times and state "Clear away all the negative thoughts, emotions and patterns that caused this (name the pattern i.e., poverty consciousness, marital abuse, alcoholism, etc.) in myself and my family". Then mentally draw a Mental/Emotional Symbol, say its name three times, then state: "Allow this change to take place within myself and my family in peace and harmony." Finally draw a Distance Symbol, say its name three times, then state: "Ensure that

all future generations of my family no longer inherit this negative pat-
tern (say the name of the pattern)". Open your eyes and take your hands
away from your solar plexus when you feel peaceful.

Malachite and Quartz

The Malachite promotes dreams of childhood problems that need resolv-
ing and the Quartz prevents the dreams from becoming nightmares and will
also begin the healing process needed. If you remember your dream in the
morning and find the problem continues to stay in your consciousness then:

Close your eyes, place your hands on your solar plexus, mentally draw
the Distance Symbol, say its name three times, then say the name of
the problem three times. Next, mentally draw a Power Symbol, say its
name three times, and state: "Clear away all the negative thoughts, emo-
tions, hurts imagined and real, and all negative patterns that have
developed from this problem." Then mentally draw a Mental/Emotional
Symbol, say its name three times, then state: "Allow this change to take
place within me and my life in peace and harmony." Open your eyes
and take your hands away from your solar plexus when you feel a sense
of peace.

Lapis Lazuli

This stone helps you to gain an inner knowing about ideas and problems and will allow you to see the truth in a given situation. It is a good stone
to place under your pillow if you are angry about something. In the morning you will know how to deal with the cause of your anger in a more positive,
but less aggressive way. You can also write down an idea or problem you
want solved on some paper and place it under your pillow with the Lapis
Lazuli. You will often wake up "knowing" the answer.

Elestial

This crystal is not a healing stone but it can be used to help receive answers
and understanding about all manner of questions. You can even ask it to
suggest what question would be best for you to ask at this time. It will often
bring into your awareness the area where you should be focusing your thoughts
and attention that will bring beneficial changes into your life. This crystal
can be placed under your pillow or you can place it with a Rose Quartz on
the desk or table where you are working.

Elestial and Purple Sapphire

These two crystals bring peace of mind, balance and a good night's sleep. However, during the following day you may have intuitive insights into many of the things that you focus on or work on. For best results it is recommended that you sleep with these two crystals under your pillow for at least five consecutive nights.

Rose Quartz and Moonstone

This combination allows you to relax and sleep deeply and peacefully.

CARRYING CRYSTALS WITH YOU

You can carry crystals on your body. You can do this by carrying them in your pockets, by tucking them into your bra (if you wear one) or wearing them as a bracelet or necklace. I found the most convenient way was to make a small bag with a long cord so I could wear it around my neck. This allowed me to try out unusual single crystals. I found that wearing the crystals had a greater effect on my body than sending their energy to me via Distance/Absent Healing did. The Distance/Absent Healing technique seemed to work more directly with the mental/emotional level. The crystals seemed to work more on the physical level when I placed them around or on my body. However, by choosing crystals that work on the mental/emotional and spiritual levels, they can be carried with you to ensure you remain serene, cheerful and confident throughout your day.

If a wound or injury is taking too long to heal or is not healing at all, place some quartz crystals around the injury with their points directed at the injury. You can either tuck them into the bandages you have around the injury or hold them in place with a Band-Aid.

CONCLUSION

Working with crystals and Reiki together is fun and I hope you enjoy it as much as I do. There are probably many more crystals that can be used with Reiki and my list is not definitive; just a beginning, an illustration of possibilities. I hope you will take time to explore and enjoy this branch of healing.

RECOMMENDED READING

There are a large number of books written about crystals. Below is a list of some that helped me to understand crystals and how to work with them.

Ananda, Vidya—*Crystals: Foundation Stones of the New World*. Universal Light Press, 1987.

Bonwitz, Ra—*Cosmic Crystals*. The Aquarian Press, 1983. (This book gives a good explanation of how the energies of crystals operate.)

Chase, Pamela Louise & Powlik, Jonathan—*The Newcastle Guide to Healing with Gemstones*. Newcastle Publishing Co. Inc., 1989.

D'Andrea, Maria—*Psychic Vibrations of Crystals, Gems & Stones*. Inter Light Publications. (This book also includes a good explanation of how to use a pendulum.)

Davis, Mikol and Lane, Earle—*Rainbows of Life*. Harper Colophon Books. (This book is about Kirlian Photography and gives a good explanation of our aura and energy fields.)

Gardner, Joy—*Color and Crystals—A Journey Through the Chakras*. The Crossing Press, 1998.

Glade, Phyllis—*Crystal Healing - The Next Step*. Llewellyn Publications, 1988.

Holbeche, Soozie—*The Power of Gems and Crystals—How they can transform your life*. Judy Piatkus (Publishers) Ltd., 1989.

Melody—*Love is in the Earth—Laying-on-of-Stones*. Earth-Love Publishing House, 1992.—*Love is in the Earth—A Kaleidoscope of Crystals—Update*. Earth-Love Publishing House, 1995.

Raphaell, Katrina—*Crystal Enlightenment Vol. 1*. Aurora Press, 1985.—*Crystal Healing Vol. 2*. Aurora Press, 1987.

Schumann, Walter—*Minerals of the World*. Sterling Publishing Co. Inc., New York.

Chapter Four...

3A Degree
Advanced Reiki

Sometimes the steps of a journey

Don't have to be as big as we imagined.

ACKNOWLEDGEMENTS

My thanks go to Reiki Master Barbara Pillsbury for taking me to the Advanced Reiki level, to Reiki Master Tina Webb who gave me Temporary Heart Attunements at her Reiki Support Group and showed me what a wonderful tool they are, and to my many Reiki friends and students who allowed me to give them Temporary Heart Attunements. I would also like to thank Reiki Practitioner Jillian McKenzie for insisting that I teach 3A Reiki Degree classes.

INTRODUCTION

The highest level or degree of Reiki is 3rd Degree. In some Reiki lineages this degree has now developed into two levels—3A, also known as Advanced Reiki, and 3rd Degree. The 3rd Degree of Reiki is often called the Reiki Master Degree and is taught to Reiki Practitioners who want to teach Reiki to others. The 3A level was developed for those people who wish to progress to the highest level of Reiki but who do not want to teach.

Degrees of Reiki

This degree originated with Barbara Weber Ray's lineage, which is known as the Radiance Technique. It came into being sometime in the 1980s, after Mrs. Takata's death, and was first known as Advanced Reiki. In Advanced Reiki students were taught a version of the Usui Reiki Master symbol and were given a different version of it when they became Reiki Masters. This often gave people an impression there were two Reiki Master symbols. The emphasis of this level of Reiki is on personal and spiritual growth.

Advanced Reiki later evolved into the 3A Degree of Reiki. During a 3A class students not only learn a version of the Usui Reiki Master symbol but they are also taught how to do a temporary heart attunement. The emphasis is still on personal and spiritual growth, but this level has also become a step towards a Master Degree of Reiki. Some Masters do not accept students to this level unless they agree to continue on to the Reiki Master level. Some lineages of Reiki have begun to refer to the 3A or Advanced Reiki level as their Reiki Master Degree and their Reiki Master level as their Reiki Teacher level.

I have found the 3A Reiki Degree useful for both those who have an inner urge to do the Reiki Master level but have a reluctance to teach or who do not feel ready to teach and those who do want to teach Reiki. It gives those Reiki Practitioners who plan on being Reiki Masters time to integrate the energy of the Usui Reiki Master symbol and practice using an attunement; making their movement into the role of Reiki Master easier.

WHY AND WHEN TO LEARN 3A (ADVANCED) REIKI

The time you spend practicing and experiencing 2nd Degree Reiki is valuable and I believe it shouldn't be rushed. You may find that many Reiki Masters have very firm ideas about how long you should wait before taking a 3rd Degree class. This time will vary from Reiki Master to Reiki Master. If you do not agree with the time you are expected to remain a 2nd Degree Reiki Practitioner before undertaking a 3A/Advanced Reiki or Reiki Master class, find a teacher who is less strict, since there is sure to be one. However, I suggest you meditate on why you want to rush through your 2nd Degree and why you want to challenge your Reiki Master on their requirements for the classes they teach.

3A Degree — Advanced Reiki

The level of 3A/Advanced Reiki is optional within the system of Reiki. Ultimately it is your choice whether you want to do this level or not. If you want to become a Reiki Master without completing this Degree you can. There are many Reiki Masters who do not teach this level and are happy for you to do Reiki Master training without you completing it. If you do want to experience this level of Reiki you may need to search for a Reiki Master who teaches it. The Reiki Masters who live in your locality are a good place to start. The Internet is another place to find information about Reiki Masters and what they teach.

You should be very familiar with your 2nd Degree Reiki symbols before attempting this Degree. Although some Reiki Masters spend time going over these symbols at the beginning of their class, not knowing your 2nd Degree symbols properly is an indication that you are not really ready to continue on to 3A/Advanced Reiki, or Reiki Master level. There is enough to learn in a 3A class without having to relearn the 2nd Degree symbols as well.

If you do want to do this level of Reiki you need to ask the Reiki Master just what it is they teach in their 3A/Advanced Reiki class. I recommend choosing a teacher who has learned and experienced this level before becoming a Reiki Master because they will have a better understanding of what you can do with this degree and what you are likely to go through as you work at this level.

Because the 3A/Advanced Reiki class has 'evolved' not all Reiki Masters teach it the same way nor do all 3A/Advanced Reiki classes contain the same content. My preference is for a class that includes:
1. An attunement to the Reiki Master Symbol.
2. The Reiki Master Symbol; how to draw it and say its name.
3. How to use the Reiki Master Symbol in treatments.
4. How to do a Temporary Heart Attunement.
5. How to send Distance Temporary Heart Attunements.
6. How to give yourself a Temporary Heart Attunement.

Degrees of Reiki

THE USUI REIKI MASTER SYMBOL

During a 3A/Advance Reiki Degree class you will be attuned to and taught how to use the fourth Reiki symbol; the Usui Reiki Master Symbol. Although this symbol has been published in several books and on the Internet there is still a strong feeling within the Reiki community that the Usui Reiki Master Symbol should not be shown or spoken about to anyone who is not a 3A/Advanced Reiki or Reiki Master practitioner. Because of this I will refer to it in this book as the Usui Reiki Master Symbol. As with the Second Degree Reiki symbols, although it is sacred, it is important to learn how to draw, say its name, and use this symbol as automatically as you use your fork and knife.

There are a number of different versions of the Usui Reiki Master Symbol around as well as non-Reiki symbols that are now used in Reiki, such as the Non-traditional Master Symbol. The Usui Reiki Master Symbol I refer to is the Japanese or Eastern Reiki version of the symbol. Its three Kanji characters can be found in a Japanese/English dictionary. Other variations of this symbol have come about because people in the Western world did not understand Japanese. Because the name of the symbol relates directly to and means the same as the Kanji characters that make up the Usui Reiki Master symbol, the name of the symbol can be used on its own. Although drawing the symbol then saying its name is the ideal, there are occasions when it is useful to just say the name of the symbol.

Drawing the Reiki Master Symbol follows the same rules that apply to drawing the Reiki Distance Symbol; horizontal lines before vertical, left strokes before right and the center stroke of a box before the bottom line of the box is closed. You should be given time in your 3A/Advance Reiki class to practice the Usui Reiki Master symbol until you can write it easily, remember it, and say the name of the symbol without difficulty.

The Reiki Master symbol can be used on its own or with any or all of the other Reiki Symbols. It can be used in any order in relation to the other Reiki symbols. The order in which you use the Reiki symbols simply determines the order in which the energies of the symbols are activated. However it is interesting to look at the symbols in the order they are usually taught. You will see they have their own innate progression.

Power Symbol	**Physical level**
Mental/Emotional Symbol	**Mental/Emotional level**
Distance Symbol	**Spiritual level**
Usui Reiki Master Symbol	**Integration of all three levels**

If a problem doesn't go away, drawing all four symbols in the above order helps.

1. Hold your hands out in the auric field about 20 inches above the body. Bring them slowly in towards the body. If you feel a resistance, draw the four Reiki Symbols in the above order (or draw the 1st two symbols and say their names three times and just say the names of the 2nd two symbols three times).
2. Continue to bring your hands slowly in towards the body. Every time you feel a resistance repeat all four symbols.
3. When your hands reach the body do all four symbols again and Reiki for as long as you intuitively feel that area needs Reiki.

Blessing

The first three strokes of the Usui Reiki Master symbol are a Kanji character that is said to have great blessing power, therefore the symbol can be used as a blessing. This can be done by mentally drawing the symbol over the receiver/client at the end of a treatment with the intent that they are blessed with their positive wishes. It can also be sent during Reiki Distance/Absent Healing as a blessing.

The Reiki Master Symbol and the 3rd level of Reiki promise to bless you with your wishes. Your wishes are your thoughts and intentions. Reiki is non-polarized energy, which means it is neither negative nor positive energy but the two combined. The spiritual level is also non-polarized. Therefore neither the level nor Reiki discriminate between right and wrong, or positive and negative. The energy will be influenced by the emotions surrounding your intents and thoughts. If you are feeling and speaking negatively then you will get a negative result. If you are feeling and speaking positively then you will get a positive result. It is expected that when you reach this level you will have mastered your thoughts and intentions so that they are always for your highest good.

Many 3A students and Reiki Masters find their lives get worse after doing a 3rd Degree class instead of better. They get sicker or unhappier. To make changes in your life you have to change how you think and speak. Instead of talking about sickness and doom and gloom you have to start thinking and talking about good things, happy times, fun things and things you are interested in and enjoy. When your words and thoughts about your life become positive at this level then life becomes magical.

Affirmations

Affirmations are a good way of training thoughts and intents to be more positive. They can be enhanced with the Reiki symbols.

1. Write the affirmation on a piece of paper. Draw all four symbols on the paper around the affirmation. Hold the paper between your hands and Reiki it.
2. Say the affirmation then mentally draw the Reiki Master symbol and say its name three times.

An affirmation needs to be repeated many times before results become noticeable. Some say affirmations should be repeated at least 15 times each day to bypass the ego.

Karma

The Healing Buddha sutra indicates that the healing energy of the universe can be used at the 3rd level to release and let go of karma—past thoughts, words and actions that are having, or will have, a negative effect on your present and future. The more you use the Usui Reiki Master symbol in your self-treatments and in your life, the less effect your past negative karma will have and the more you will generate positive karma for a fortunate future.

21 Day Self Treatments

It is highly recommended that 3A/Advanced Reiki Practitioners do 21 days of self-treatments, after their class, using only the Reiki Master symbol at each hand position during the treatments. This helps you over the healing crisis, allowing you to integrate the three levels, and also experience and recognize the energy of the Reiki Master symbol. You can use the other Reiki symbols at any other time of the day, but it seems to be important to just use the Reiki Master symbol for 21 days in your self-treatments after a 3rd Degree attunement.

3A Degree — Advanced Reiki

I have been approached on a number of occasions by Reiki students who have done their 3A/Advanced class (especially when it is called a Reiki Master class) with lineages where 21 Day self-treatments were never mentioned. They have said they were in a mess and out of balance since doing their 3rd level class. They often think it is because something was wrong with the Master or how the Master attuned them. I recommended that they do a 21-day self treatment using the Reiki Master symbol only and this has brought them back into balance again.

There are a number of ways you can draw the Reiki Master symbol at each hand position. For example:

- Draw the symbol on the palms of your hands before placing them on yourself.
- Draw the symbol sideways on the front body positions and press it into the body with your hands.
- Mentally draw the symbol and tell it to go to the hand position you are about to do.
- Draw the Usui Reiki Master Symbol at the beginning of your self-treatment and then just mentally repeat the name of the symbol at each hand position as many times as you like.

Used regularly the Reiki Master symbol has an enormous capacity to empower and promote mental/emotional and spiritual growth and physical healing.

THE TEMPORARY HEART ATTUNEMENT

There are several different Reiki attunement techniques in use in the Reiki community. All of them are effective. Usually the first attunement of the 'four attunements' of 1st Degree Reiki that Mrs. Takata and early Western Reiki Masters taught is used for the Temporary Heart Attunement. Your Reiki Master will teach the attunement he/she knows during your class. As we always choose the 'right Reiki Master' the attunement you are taught will also be the 'right attunement for you' even though it may be different to another Reiki Practitioner's attunement.

The attunement process is a formula, which with practice, becomes easy to do. It is also a sacred spiritual initiation that connects the receiver/client with the higher levels of consciousness that connect to the 'God' level of the universe. Reiki is a gift that comes directly from the highest spiritual source. It should always be treated with the greatest respect. Many people receiving an attunement find it a very profound moment in their lives. I recommend that you always treat the Reiki attunement, regardless of whether it is temporary or not, as a special, spiritual experience. With that attitude, I believe, you will gain in personal growth from each attunement you give.

Whoever you give a Reiki attunement to, always treat that person as special and give the attunement as professionally as you can. Make the place where you give an attunement a special place and the attunement a special event; play relaxing music or maybe light a candle.

Reiki Guides

Having Reiki Guides was a shock for me when I did the 3rd level of Reiki. I had no idea there were such beings and when my Master asked me which ones I wanted to work with I wasn't sure I wanted anyone. It took me a while to get used to the idea. Eventually I learned to trust them and to enjoy working with them.

You need to think and meditate about the Higher Beings you want to work with at this level. The following are the Buddhist names of the Higher Beings who work with Reiki:

Vajrapani	Thunder-bolt-in-the-hands	Power Symbol
Padmapani (Avalokitesvara)	Lotus-in-the-hands	Mental / Emotional Symbol
Manjushri	Bodhisattva of Wisdom	Distance Symbol
Dainichi	Great Sun	Reiki Master Symbol
Ko Myo	Light of the Sun & Moon	Reiki Master Symbol
Gakko	Bodhisattva Light of the Moon	Reiki Master Symbol
Nikko	Bodhisattva Light of the Sun	Reiki Master / Distance Symbols
Vajradhara	Thunderbolt King (Great Mother)	Reiki Master Symbol
Healing Buddha	Master of Healing	Reiki Master Symbol

Reiki Practitioners have worked with the spirit and energies of Jesus Christ, all the various Angels and Archangels, Ascended Reiki Masters, and their own Spiritual Guides. My recommendation for 3A/Advanced Reiki students is to pick just one or two guides and work with them a few times before adding others. Or you can experiment by choosing a different guide each time you do an attunement until you find those you like working with. I also believe that Reiki gives you special Reiki/healing guides. You may become aware of them during the class or after you have done several attunements. Sometimes it will be the person receiving the attunement who becomes aware of your guides and tells you about them. The more you work with your guides the more relaxed you will become about them and the sooner you will build a relationship with them based on trust. You can do this by giving regular attunements to yourself and others and starting each day thanking your guides and asking them to help and protect you throughout the day.

I feel it is necessary that you know and understand that you are just channeling the attunement just as you channel Reiki when you give a treatment, otherwise your ego can become inflated and misled with self-importance. The work you do during an attunement is symbolic. The hand positions and symbols used in the attunement give permission for the energy channels to be opened and for the receiver to be tuned to Reiki. The actual attuning to the energy is done in the unseen realms where your guides reside.

The knowledge that there are guides to help you with a Reiki attunement can give you confidence. You can ask for help from your guides if you forget or get stuck during an attunement. The person receiving the attunement will not mind if the attunement takes a little longer because you stopped a moment to mentally ask your guides for help. Often the person receiving the attunement has no idea what is going to happen in it so they don't notice the time taken or the moments when you hesitate.

The 3A level of Reiki is also a level of practice and experimentation. The more practice and experimenting you do at this level, the easier it will be for you to do your Reiki Master/Teacher training.

A Temporary Self-Attunement

3A Reiki Practitioners can give themselves a temporary self-attunement. You can use a temporary self-attunement for healing, to give yourself more energy, or to implant a powerful intent (always remembering the intent will only be activated by Reiki if it is in tune with the goodness and healing of Reiki).

It seems to me that there are differences between the various methods for temporary self-attunements. I use the surrogate method (a doll) to help get rid of headaches, or other aches and pains, while the one I do on my knees I find to be very uplifting and harmonizing when I am tired or feeling a bit down about something. The mirror image method tends to take me off into another consciousness where I feel a bit 'spaced out'.

Self-Attunement On Yourself

This attunement is done while seated. The Reiki Practitioner's knees, thighs and non-dominant hand are used as witness for the attunement. For example:

Right knee	represents	the back of your head
Right thigh	represents	your back
Left knee	represents	the front of your head
Left thigh	represents	the front of your body
Non-dominant hand	represents	both hands

In your preparation for the attunement state that it will be for you and what parts of your body will be represented by your knees and thighs then proceed with the Temporary Heart Attunement.

Self-Attunement Using a Surrogate (doll, teddy bear or pillow).

This attunement is done on a doll, bear or pillow. Place the surrogate in a chair and do the Temporary Heart Attunement on it as though it is a real person. During the preparation section of your attunement say that the attunement is for you.

Self Attunement on Your Image In a Mirror

You can also give yourself a self-attunement by sitting in front of a mirror and doing the Temporary Heart Attunement formula on your image.

Distance/Absent Temporary Attunement

You can send a Temporary Heart Attunement to someone who is not with you. Known as a Distance or Absent Temporary Heart Attunement, it seems to be more effective when the person receiving it is told what time it will be done and then asked to sit in a quiet, meditative state during that time.

Once you have prepared yourself for an attunement draw the Distance Symbol, say its name three times, say the name of the person you are sending the attunement to and then proceed with the rest of the attunement by doing it:
1. on your knees, thighs and non-dominant hand, or
2. on a surrogate—usually a doll, teddy bear or pillow, or
3. on a visualization/image of the person sitting in a chair, or
4. on a photo of the person.

Healing Attunement

The Temporary Heart Attunement can be used as a healing attunement before or after a Reiki Treatment. I personally like to use it before a Reiki Treatment as it helps to relax the receiver/client and begins the healing process before the treatment actually starts. The Temporary Heart Attunement is often given after someone has had a series of treatments to enable them to continue giving themselves Reiki until their next treatment or until they are able to take a 1st Degree Reiki class.

I heard that giving a series of Temporary Heart Attunements to people with epilepsy was helpful. With the agreement of a friend who has epilepsy, I decided to experiment. This person was having trouble with voices telling her terrible things and giving her horrible visions. I gave her Distance/Absent Temporary Attunements every evening for 21 days. The voices stopped and the visions disappeared. One of her last visions was of Christ, dressed in blue, holding out his arms to her. Her doctor reduced the medication that had been affecting her speech and which made her feel drowsy and lifeless. The next time I met her she was sparkling with energy, was happy and enjoying her life and feeling balanced. I have also successfully done a series of Distance/Absent Temporary Attunements on a woman suffering from frequent migraines and depression, and on another person who was finding life a struggle, with good results.

When I originally gave a series of Temporary Heart Attunements, I committed myself to doing them every day for 21 days. However, after the first 14 days I struggled to remember to do the attunements. Now I find that 14 days of Distance/Absent Temporary Heart Attunements followed by daily Distance/Absent Healing for a couple of months works best.

Attuning Plants, Animals, etc.

You can do Temporary Heart Attunements on plants, animals, stones, crystals and inanimate objects. Try doing an attunement on your potted plants and see the response. Animals may not stand still long enough but you can attune them by using a Distance/Absent Temporary Attunement. Some people like to attune crystals, rocks and shells that they have placed around their homes. You can attune your car, boat or other equipment for protection and to ensure good performance and longevity.

Attuning Specific Parts of the Body

During a Temporary Heart Attunement you can give an attunement to specific parts of the body such as the eyes, throat, knees, feet, elbows, etc. Attuning a specific part of the body is usually done when there is an injury, discomfort or pain in a particular area. It can help kick start the healing process for a chronic illness or an injury that isn't healing. The attunement provides a large boost of energy to accelerate healing.

When one part of the body is injured or not well its pair will be under stress as it tries to do the work of both. If the part of the body that you are going to attune is one of a pair then attune both parts so that they remain in balance i.e., attune both knees, feet, eyes, kidneys, lungs, etc.

Foot Attunement

Attuning feet has been popular from time to time within the Reiki community. It has been said that attuning feet will help you to walk your spiritual journey and enables you to give Reiki to the earth as you walk and so on. However, I personally have not noticed anything in particular happen except that it was a very pleasant attunement at the time. Attuning feet is an example of doing an attunement on a specific part of the body.

1. Do your Temporary Heart Attunement up to the point where you have finished blowing on the hands.
2. Instead of finishing off the attunement the next step is to sit or kneel on the floor in front of the receiver/client. Lift up the foot that is nearest to you, so it is easy for you to work with it. You can either

rest their foot on your knee or support the heel of their foot in your non-dominant hand—use whichever is more comfortable.

3. To attune the foot draw the symbols, in the same order as you did for the hands, a few inches away from the sole of the foot so you do not tickle the person receiving the attunement. Press each symbol gently into the sole as you say its name three times.

4. Do the blow technique, like you would normally do after attuning the hands, from the top of the foot to the heel of the foot and back up to the toes again.

5. Place their foot back onto the floor. Shift your position so you can attune the other foot.

6. When the second foot is attuned, stand up and complete the rest of the attunement.

Demonstrating Reiki

The temporary Heart Attunement is useful for those people who wish to 'try before they buy' so it is sometimes used to demonstrate what being attuned to Reiki is like. It gives a person the opportunity to experience Reiki before making the decision to attend a 1st Degree Reiki class.

It is recommended that you do the attunement in a private rather than a public area where there may be people who are hostile to, afraid of, or misunderstand initiations and attunements. Also, the attunement is a sacred experience and it is hard to create a special atmosphere and space in a crowd.

Time Factor

The Heart Attunement is temporary. It can last from approximately one week to eight weeks. On rare occasions it has been known to last for three months. The length of time the attunement is effective is dependent on the receiver/client; how often they use Reiki, and how open they are to receiving the attunement. The receiver/client does not need to believe in Reiki for it to work, but he/she does need to believe in it to use it. If they have a resistance to the idea of Reiki, or a disbelief in your ability to do Reiki, it may not last long because they will not like using it. If a person is open to the idea of Reiki and enjoys using the energy, they will be able to do Reiki for a longer period of time.

The person giving a temporary Reiki attunement is not responsible for the length of time it lasts. Before you give someone a Temporary Heart Attunement always tell the receiver/client that it is a temporary attunement and it will be effective from approximately one week to a month. It is better to underestimate the length of time it will be effective rather than overestimate.

The Experience of Giving an Attunement

When giving a Temporary Reiki Attunement you may experience the energy of Reiki differently for each person you attune. With some receivers/clients you may not feel the energy at all. With others you will feel it as a very spiritual and profound occasion, or you may simply feel the energy flow in a similar way as it does during a treatment. The receiver/client will draw through Reiki as they need it.

Whatever you may feel, trust Reiki and your spiritual assistants. They do know what they are doing. Continue the whole attunement, then ask the receiver/client what they experienced. Just as Reiki works every time you give a Reiki treatment, the same happens when you do an attunement.

I usually do most of an attunement with my eyes closed because I experience the energy as light in my mind's eye. I see the light sometimes as pure white, or as tiny rainbows streaming down into a receiver/client, or as yellow edged in orange, or as red light. Sometimes I see nothing at all. I like to feel the energy flow through me as I channel it into the receiver/client so I do not race through an attunement but try to flow with the process in unity with the energy flow. During an attunement I get thoughts and ideas that I follow. For instance: instructions to place my hands on a particular part of the body such as knees or feet or to hold my hands for a longer time in one of the attunement hand positions. Sometimes the thought is an affirmation or intention. When this happens I do what my thoughts have suggested to me.

The Sacredness of an Attunement

The Reiki attunement is sacred because it works with the energies of 'God' (also known as 'All that Is' or the creative power of the Universe). If you start an attunement ALWAYS finish it. Don't stop to do something else during an attunement. If the phone rings, let it ring. If you get a tickle in your throat mentally clear it with a Power Symbol not a glass of water. Don't chat to someone who is giving or receiving an attunement and don't chat while you are giving an attunement. From the time you begin asking your guides to assist with the attunement the place where you and the receiver(s) are, becomes sacred or spiritual—a special place that belongs to 'God'.

If you are giving an attunement to a group of people ask, before you start, that they stay seated until everyone has received their attunement and you have said thank you.

Giving an Attunement to One or More People

Attunements are usually given to one person at a time. The person sits in a chair while you do a complete attunement on them. If you have several people to give attunements to you can do them one at a time so that when one attunement is completed the receiver/client will get out of the chair and another person will take their place. You can also give attunements to a group of people sitting on chairs in a circle or in a line. The group can be as big as you like. However, some people do get fidgety and bored sitting still for a long period of time. An attunement takes about 2 to 5 minutes to do depending on how fast you do the attunement. If you have twenty people it will mean they will be sitting without talking or much movement for 40 to 100 minutes. Many people cannot sit still and be quiet for that length of time. I have found 12 people are the most I like to attune in one group. Three groups of four people in each are better, because two groups can go outside or into another room and chat while one group receives an attunement. Personally I like receiving attunements as a member of a large circle because I can stay in the attunement energy for much longer than you would normally do in a single attunement.

When I attune people sitting in a circle I do the complete attunement on a person before moving on to the next person. If I have them sitting in a line I have a choice of doing the whole attunement before moving on to the next person or I can go down one side of the row doing the first part of the attunement and then walk to the other side of the row and go down that side doing the next part of the attunement and so on until the whole attunement is completed.

As a 3A Reiki Practitioner it is good to be able to experiment with the various ways of doing attunements i.e., one person at a time, a group in a circle facing the center, a group in a circle facing outwards, or as a group sitting in a line of chairs. It you attend a Reiki Support Group ask if anyone wants to have a Temporary Heart Attunement before they give and receive treatments. Or arrange for members of the group to receive them at another time during the week. This will give you plenty of opportunities to practice attunements on others.

THE PROCESS OF 3A DEGREE REIKI

I believe that the 3rd level of Reiki requires a significant integration of the energy. This level is the spiritual level and to work in this level requires balance and harmony between the physical and mental/emotional levels. If the Reiki Practitioner has not done enough work at the previous degrees of Reiki, they may find that they need to do a lot of work to bring themselves into balance and wellness at the 3rd level. Many people have little or no experience of the spiritual level and are often skeptical or afraid of it. Consequently they can experience profound shifts at the 3rd level of Reiki regardless of whether they enter this level during a 3A, Advanced Reiki or Reiki Master class.

The Usui Reiki Master symbol allows us to integrate all three levels of Reiki and also opens doorways safely into the invisible/intangible/spiritual world around us. The attunement process allows us to work in and with the healing energy of that world that we call Reiki, which can be interpreted as Spiritual Life Force Energy.

The Healing Crisis

Most Reiki Practitioners will have experienced some kind of healing crisis prior to attending a 3A/Advanced Reiki Class. If they have not, this class will trigger one.

The attunement to the 3rd level of Reiki also seems to affect the frequency of Reiki and this can also have an effect on the Reiki Practitioner. The Reiki energy is a light wave frequency that acts in a similar way as the flow of currents in the sea. When a current changes, or is increased, there is a certain amount of turbulence at the point of change. A similar thing can happen when you change the frequency of Reiki (i.e., go to another Degree of Reiki). You may already have noticed this shortly after your 1st and 2nd Degree classes when you went through a period of adjustment. Some people refer to this period of adjustment after an attunement as a healing crisis.

There is often an increase in the pace of life after a 3A Degree attunement. I personally found the increase was simply a clearing up and cleaning out of unfinished business—things that I had allowed to drift or had not finished or had meant to get around to at some stage. I found the attunement gave me the energy, impetus and an urgency to complete these things.

Doing your 21 days of self treatments, using the Usui Master Symbol at each hand position, will give you the energy to cope with this clearing out and finishing off stage, and will bring in all that is necessary for you to re-organize your life in better ways.

Intent and Outcome

As you progress through the Reiki Degrees the use of intent becomes more important. It is recommended that you practice using affirmations as a way of learning to use intents clearly and simply. Remember it is the intent that is important not the outcome. As you work in partnership with Reiki it is your job to provide the intent and Reiki's job to provide the outcome. When a Reiki Practitioner gets fixated on the outcome they may get 'put off' Reiki because an outcome provided by Reiki is not always the outcome they anticipate or expect.

The Latin root of the word 'intend' means to 'stretch forward'. An intent (the noun of intend) produces an energy that attracts change because it stretches into the future and 'feels' a result in advance without defining a pathway or outcome to that result. This allows opportunities for the best solutions to form in the imagination and then manifest in your life. Using your will forces energy to go in one limited, controlled direction that bypasses intuition. Forcing or willing a result can be a huge waste of energy because although you may get what you want, you will probably not be satisfied by it.

You can add an intention to a Reiki treatment, during Distance/Absent Healing and while doing your preparation at the beginning of a Temporary Heart Attunement. Intent can enhance an attunement or direct it to a specific part of the body or be used to increase spiritual, physical and mental/emotional well being. You should try to accompany your intents with feelings of love or joy.

THE SPIRITUAL LEVEL

Spiritual—What is it?

Many people talk about being spiritual but sometimes do not know what the word actually means. According to the Collins English Dictionary spiritual means:
1. relating to the spirit or soul not to physical nature or matter; intangible; relating to sacred things i.e., church, religion, etc.
2. standing in relationship between souls or minds of persons involved.
3. having a mind or emotions of a high and delicately refined quality.
4. an Afro American religious song.

The Reiki Master symbol appears to allow you to safely enter the area of soul, spirit and the intangible. Before developing your spiritual level you need to work to ensure your first two levels are healed and in balance. This ensures you have a stable foundation from which to experience the 3rd level. The spiritual level requires a marriage between the physical and mental/emotional levels before it can truly come into view. In legends and fairy tales, the spiritual level is alluded to when the hero (physical (male) level) marries the princess (mental/emotional (female) level). Together they live happily ever after. When both levels come together in love and equality it creates happiness and blessings in your life. Once married the hero and princess become King and Queen and live a life of richness and ease.

Because the word spiritual means 'belonging to God' it encompasses all the things we accredit to God such as good fortune, luck, happiness, ease of living, feeling special, being talented, being a hero, as well as the things we have no control over such as the weather. God is sometimes seen as an angry or vengeful God and so we also accredit bad luck, disasters, natural justice, and problems we cannot overcome to God.

You can often tell when an illness or problem is affecting the spiritual level by the proverbs, sayings and catchwords that a person uses to describe their illness. For example: *"It's in the hands of God"* or *"it's my bad luck"* or *"this is the cross I have to bear"* or *"fate is against me"* or *"this is my karma"*, and so on. When working with someone who includes one or more of these sayings in their everyday speech you need to use the Reiki Master Symbol, followed by the Power Symbol to clear away these beliefs while you give them Reiki Treatments.

The spiritual becomes apparent to us when our soul is involved. The movement of your soul can bring moments of profound bliss and joy as well as a connectedness to, and compassion for, all living beings. These moments are amazing gifts of healing and insight on how to be truly you. When the soul is touched there is often an accompanying feeling of coming home and recognition that you are special and loved.

Spiritual Growth

At the 3rd Degree level Reiki Practitioners may find themselves becoming more intuitive, or they may have more co-incidences and pre-cognitive experiences, or have a greater awareness or interest in spiritual and religious matters; or a sense of being connected to all life; and feel the need to express who they really are as their need for truth and truthfulness increases.

The spiritual level lets you experience the richness and abundance of life on earth; it allows you to appreciate all that you are blessed with. It also lets you walk along your life path with ease. When things are not easy in your life you will find that either your physical or mental/emotional levels are out of balance. If your physical level is out of balance you could be eating the wrong things, not doing enough exercise, not getting enough sleep, too hot, too cold, not well. If your mental/emotional level is out of balance you could be thinking the wrong things, have the wrong ideas, be blaming other people, angry, worried, grieving, not interested in what you are doing. At these times you need to go back to giving yourself Reiki self-treatments to bring your physical level into balance and using the 2nd Degree Symbols to help bring your mental/emotional level back to being satisfied with who you are so you can see the good and God in others.

When your body and mind/emotions are working together you will find it easy to be happy and time will flow by without you noticing. This can be achieved by thinking about what you are doing at the time you are doing it. When you chop firewood you think about chopping firewood. When you paint a picture you think about painting the picture; don't think about what your next-door-neighbor or lover is doing. When your mind is off somewhere else while you are working or doing something physical then you will find time drags, you are likely to not do the work well or have an accident, and you will be bored with what you are doing.

Judgment can block the process of integrating the physical and mental/emotional levels and therefore can block you from reaching the spiritual level. You will have trouble focusing on what you are doing if you begin a job by saying, *"this is an awful job;"* or *"I can't do this"* or *"I don't know how to do this."* We all make these kinds of judgments everyday about work, food, people and experiences. Worry, fear, anger and indecision block the spiritual level. They also block our ability to focus on what we are doing. Repeating the Five Reiki Principles at each hand position during self-treatments can help dissolve those blocks.

FACILITATOR OF A REIKI SUPPORT GROUP

If you haven't done so before at 1st or 2nd Degree, when you reach the 3A level of Reiki give some thought to, and if possible, set up a Reiki Support Group in your area and act as a facilitator for the group. It will help to build your confidence in talking about Reiki and handling groups of people, and will benefit you should you decide to do the Reiki Master Degree. A Reiki Support Group can be a great way to meet other Reiki people and gives those attending an opportunity to practice Reiki, discuss it and enjoy a treatment. Members of your Reiki Support Group may want to be your first 2nd or 3A Degree students when you become a Reiki Master. If they enjoy your support group they will recommend you to friends and family who are looking for a Reiki Master with whom to do a 1st Degree Reiki class.

There are various kinds of support groups. They have evolved to suit the people attending them. Support groups change over time depending on the people attending, what interests them, what Reiki lineage they belong to, and who their Reiki Master or Masters were. Support groups change too because some people attend every meeting, some come occasionally, some come once and never again. They also change because the facilitator moves away from the area or hands the leadership of the group over to someone else.

If you intend to hold a Reiki Support Group here are some suggestions that are worth considering.
1. Accept each person as they are. Not everyone is as perfect as you are.
2. Don't criticize people for not attending. It is their choice. If you want to make certain people are going to turn up for a Support Group telephone them the night before to check whether they will be coming or not; but don't pressure them to attend.
3. Welcome new members. This helps to ensure your group continues, and remains fresh and interesting.

The Structure of a Support Group

When you start something it is a good idea to have a plan or outline of what you intend to do. Plans are good places to get started, but be prepared to change your plan or outline as you go along. If you decide to start a Reiki Support Group take a little time to decide what you want from it. Do you just want to receive Reiki treatments or do you want more? If so what?

Receiving and Giving Reiki Treatments.

If you just want to give and receive Reiki treatments, all you need is a massage table and a few Reiki friends.
1. Set a date and time to hold the support group. Tell your Reiki friends and put an advertisement in your local newspaper. There are usually quite a few people around who would love to attend a support group but don't know where one is being held in their locality.
2. Have a place where the group will meet i.e., your home or local church or community hall, etc. If you hold the support group at a venue that has to be paid for then work out how much it will cost each person to attend. You will need to estimate how many will attend and find an average i.e., Cost of venue is $25 per evening and you expect to have 5 to 10 people come along. You can charge everyone $4 each. If 10 people come along you will collect $40; $25 for the cost of the hall and $15 to go into your support group

fund. However, the next week if only 5 people come along you will collect $20; this will mean you have to take $5 from your support group fund to help pay the cost of the venue.

3. Decide whether you want to have tea/coffee and biscuits/cookies after the support session. If you do, decide who is going to pay for it. In many groups the tea, coffee, milk and sugar is provided by whoever is hosting the group and members of the support group take turns to provide the biscuits/cookies. If you have a support group fund you can deduct the cost of tea/coffee and biscuits from the fund.

4. Record keeping, even for a small group, can be important.

   a. **Funds**—If you have a support group fund to pay for a venue, tea, coffee, etc., keep proper records so that other members of the group can look at them if they want. This will prevent any annoyances arising about being charged for attending a Reiki Support Group when you can show people what the money is being used for.

   b. **Attendance**—It is a good idea to keep an attendance book for all those people who come along to your support group. My suggestion is to give everyone their own page so it will be easy for the information to be photocopied if someone needs to provide proof of how many hours they have spent giving/receiving Reiki or how often and frequently they have been attending a Reiki Support Group. If asked for a written reference about someone's attendance you will be able to see at a glance how often someone has come along to your group. You can also use the book when you phone or email people to remind them of the date of your next support group.

   At the top of the page write their full name, address, telephone and fax numbers, and email address. Divide the rest of the page into columns for recording the date of the support group, and signature of the Reiki Practitioner. If you wish you can record how many treatments took place and the average length of time for each treatment. Get the people attending a Support Group to sign the book when they first arrive or while they are having a cup of tea or coffee. Make it the same time at each support group meeting and then it will become a habit and won't be forgotten.

3A Degree — Advanced Reiki

Most support groups last about 2 to 3 hours. Treatment times are usually determined by the time set aside for treatments and the number of people attending i.e., 2 hours (120 minutes) divided by 6 people (20 minutes) less about 5 minutes between treatments to change over = approximately 15 minutes treatment time per person.

A Reiki Support Group that is More than just Giving and Receiving Treatments

A support group can be anything you want it to be. You can add more to it depending on what you want. Some of the groups I have attended have included meditation, energy circles, Distance/Absent Healing, a short reading followed by discussion, and an opportunity for everyone attending to say briefly what they have been doing with Reiki and how Reiki has been working in their lives since the last group meeting.

In a group such as this you need to have a facilitator or leader who will ensure that the support group follows the structure or plan that has been set for it. The more you fit into a evening the more critical timing becomes. The facilitator's main role is to ensure that all the things planned for the evening get done. Here is an example of a more structured Reiki Support Group:

1. Have all the participants seated in a circle (if possible).
2. The Group facilitator opens the evening with an introduction and welcomes everyone, with a special welcome to any newcomers.
3. If there are newcomers to the Group, ask each person in the circle to give a brief introduction of themselves that includes their name, Reiki degree, who they trained with, what they are doing with Reiki or what they love about Reiki.
4. Then spend a short time—about 15 minutes discussing what was brought forward by the group during the introduction.
5. Next the facilitator can lead a short guided-meditation—this is often optional and will depend on whether the facilitator likes doing guided meditations.
6. The facilitator can then lead the whole circle in 10—15 minutes of Reiki Distance/Absent Healing.
   a. A pad and pen are sent around the circle for everyone to write down the names of the people they want to send Distance/Absent Healing to. Alternatively, people can fill in this list when they first arrive.

b. The facilitator mentally draws the Distance Healing Symbol and asks that Reiki from the group is sent to everyone whose names are on the list.

c. Either the facilitator or someone else reads all the names aloud and then the paper is usually placed in the center of the circle. Alternatively each person can speak aloud the name or names of the people they want Distance/Absent Healing sent to.

d. First Degree Practitioners can use intent for their Reiki to assist with the Distance/Absent Healing. Second and Third Degree Practitioners can draw the Distance Healing Symbol and use their knees or fingertips to activate the flow of energy. Distance/Absent Healing will work in a group without everyone using the Distance Symbol but using it adds more energy, protection and clarity and it is a good opportunity for the Second Degree Practitioners to practice using the symbol.

7. Hold an energy circle.

a. Stand or sit in a circle and hold hands. I was taught that everyone's thumbs should point left. This means your right hand is on top of your neighbor-on-the-right's left hand and your left hand is under your neighbor-on-the-left's right hand. Why? I don't really know. It has been explained to me that it helps to guide the energy around the circle. I have found that the energy will travel around the circle no matter how you hold your hands.

b. The facilitator draws Reiki down through his/her crown to his/her heart and then mentally directs it down their left arm, through their left hand to the person on their left.

c. Each person in the circle visualizes the energy entering their right hand, travelling up their arm and across into the heart. At this point they add their love and compassion to the energy then they visualize Reiki travelling on down their left arm and into the hand of the person on their left.

d. Continue sending the energy around the circle for a minimum of two or more minutes.

e. To finish the circle the facilitator can chant the Five Reiki Principles (with everyone joining in) and then gently squeeze the hands he/she is holding and let them go.

8. The rest of the session is then taken up with giving and receiving Reiki Treatments. During these treatments each person will either keep their hands in one place on the body or change hand positions several times. Members of the group usually change where they stand at the table when the person on the table changes. Because the person who has just come off the table may feel a little 'spaced-out' they usually do the head positions for the first treatment after theirs so they can sit down. Once again the length of treatments will depend on how many people there are, how many tables you will use and how long you have to do the treatments i.e., 12 people and 3 tables = 4 people per table divided into 90 minutes would usually mean each person received a 20 minute treatment; either all done on the front of the person or 10 minutes on their front and 10 minutes on their back.

9. Finish the evening with a cup of tea/coffee and a chat.

Reiki Support Groups can include time for learning new techniques about Reiki. You can do this by allowing the people in your group to share how they use Reiki. Or you can practice the hand positions described in the book *The Original Reiki Handbook of Dr. Mikao Usui*, or explore some of the ideas described in other Reiki books, other alternative healing modalities and spiritual books.

CONCLUSION

The 3A level allows the step from 2nd Degree to 3rd Degree to be easier and gives you time to integrate and experience Reiki at the third level before facing the world and taking on the full mantle of Reiki Master. It gives you time to experiment and have fun with the Reiki Master symbol and experience the attunement process without the expectations that you and the world have about being a Reiki Master. It is a time to simply enjoy using Reiki. It is also a time to explore whether you do want to take on the responsibility of the Master role. Many people find the 3A/Advanced Reiki level satisfying and find they no longer have an internal feeling of being 'pushed' to be a Reiki Master. For them it is more important to work with themselves at the third level of Reiki than to teach Reiki to others.

For others the experience of the 3A/Advanced Reiki level confirms their inner intuition that their pathway is to teach Reiki. Running a support group and giving temporary attunements enables them to explore interacting with groups of people and with passing on attunements to others.

RECOMMENDED READING

Petter, Frank Arjava and Usui, Dr. Mikao—*The Original Reiki Handbook of Dr. Mikao Usui.* Published by Lotus Press, PO Box 325, Twin Lakes, WI 53181, USA, 1999.

Two books about nutrition that I found very helpful are:

D'Adamo, Peter J. Dr.—*Eat Right for Your Type.* Published by Century Books Limited, Random House UK Ltd., 20 Vauxhall Bridge Rd., London SW1V 2SA, UK, 2001.

Weissberg, Steven M. and Christiano, Joseph—*The Answer is in Your Bloodtype.* Published by Personal Nutrition USA, Inc.

Many people have written about the spiritual level. For example:

Adrienne, Carol—*The Purpose of Your Life.* Published by Eagle Books, William Morrow and Company Inc., 1350 Avenue of the Americas, New York, NY 10019, USA, 1998.

O'Donohue, John—*Anam Cara Spiritual Wisdom from The Celtic World.* Published by Bantam Books, Great Britain, 1997.

Zukav, Gary—*Soul Stories.* Published by Simon & Schuster UK Ltd., Africa Huse, 64-78 Kingsway, London WC2B 6AH, England, 2000.

Books on legends and fairy tales are interesting to read. Many of them are stories about the spiritual level. For example:

The Twelve Princesses—this is a story about how you spend your time when you are sleeping; your physical level (the 12 princes) and your mental/emotional level (the 12 princesses) dance together and enjoy themselves. The soldier (ego who discovers where they go and what they do) marries one of the princesses (intuition). The 12 princesses also represent 12 hours. He marries the youngest princess who symbolizes the present hour i.e., he keeps his mind in the present and lives happily ever after (the spiritual level).

Each legend and fairy tale reaffirms that our physical and mental/emotional levels must fall in love and enjoy being together for us to be happy, fulfilled and in tune with the spiritual level of life. The more you read these stories the more likely you will see deeper meanings within them. They are designed to reach into the archetypal regions of the mind where their message can trigger a deeper understanding of life and living.

Chapter Five...

3rd Degree Reiki Master & Teacher

Just when you think the journey is over

You begin again at a different level.

A journey, within a journey, within a journey.

The Master journey, within the Reiki journey,

within Life's journey.

ACKNOWLEDGEMENTS

*M*y thanks go to Reiki Master Barbara Pillsbury who took me through my 3rd Degree Reiki Training, to Reiki Masters Bobbe Free and Elizabeth Currey for their Master extension class, to all the Reiki Masters I have met at classes, gatherings, retreats and on the Internet. Thank you for your examples as Reiki Masters and for the discussions we've had about Reiki and the Reiki Master level. My thanks also go to the Reiki Masters I have trained, for you have all taught me so much.

REIKI MASTER

INTRODUCTION

Traditionally there were only three degrees of Reiki; 1st, 2nd and Reiki Master. The Reiki Master level was taught to people who were fully committed to teaching Reiki. The fees of Reiki Master training were out of reach for many ensuring that only the very well-to-do or the very determined became Reiki Masters. Eventually the price structure for Reiki training was challenged and Reiki is now taught at a varying range of prices within reach of most people. This has enabled some people to do the Reiki Master level without making a commitment to teaching Reiki; instead opting to experience the Master level for themselves and their own personal growth.

WHEN, WHY AND HOW TO BECOME A REIKI MASTER

There are many opinions about when someone is ready to become a Reiki Master. It is my personal opinion that the energy we call Reiki will send you a feeling, a sign, or a series of coincidences to indicate it is time to move to this level.

The Reiki Master level, like the other degrees of Reiki, requires a Reiki attunement/initiation. You can supplement your training by reading books about Reiki, but you will not become a Reiki Master just by reading books. You must go to a Reiki Master to be attuned to this level. You have the right to decide who does your Reiki Master training. Many Reiki Masters conduct interviews with potential Reiki Master students, others have questionnaires to be filled in, and some accept whoever comes along and pays the fee. Some Reiki Masters will only teach you this level if you attend 1st and 2nd Degree again with them, while others will accept your previous Reiki training and just teach you the Reiki Master level. The requirements Reiki Masters set to determine whom they will teach at this level is their choice. If you don't like their criteria then find another Master. Arguing with a Reiki Master about what they should or should not teach and what they should or should not charge indicates you probably will have little respect for what and how they teach, and that you will not enjoy a Master/student relationship with that Master.

You can choose the same Master that you did one or more of your previous degrees with or you can choose someone different. It is neither compulsory nor are you obligated to do all your Reiki degrees with the same Master. Choose someone you get along well with because your relationship with your Reiki Master can often extend beyond your training period and it is a bonus if that relationship turns into a mutual friendship of equals. It is also easier to learn from someone you respect and admire.

Every Reiki Master, I believe, is entitled to decide what fees to charge for Reiki training. Fees can be a point of contention and resentment for some and you really don't need to bring those negative thoughts and feelings into your Reiki Master training. Let them go. If you do not like the fees a Master charges, find another Reiki Master who charges fees that you are happy with. There are plenty of people available these days who can teach Reiki so shop around and find someone who suits you.

Asking a Reiki Master if you can pay off your Reiki Master fees slowly over a long period of time is, as far as I am concerned, unfair. Mrs. Takata is reputed to have said, *"For Reiki Master you should mortgage your house."* I believe this means you should get a loan from the bank to pay your Reiki Master fees and arrange with the bank to pay the loan off as it suits you. Most Reiki Masters do not have the expertise to formulate loan contracts or the financial backing to extend unlimited credit or pay back time to their students—banks do.

In the past it was said that *'when the student was ready the money would be available'*. This inferred that money and spiritual readiness went hand-in-hand. This opinion appeared to be supported to some degree by the mythical story of Mikao Usui's experiences in the Beggar City. Once it was discovered that the Reiki Story was not factual this opinion began to lose favor, especially with people who feel that money detracts from spiritual life. I believe that because our feelings about money can be very strong those feelings often act as a guideline to whether we are travelling on our right pathway. The resentment felt about paying a certain sum for a Reiki class may actually indicate more than just the price being too high. Your feelings may indicate that you don't really want to learn Reiki from that particular Master or to learn that form of Reiki. People with good friends who become Reiki Masters sometimes have difficulty paying fees to them because it requires them to adjust their view of the friendship and to sometimes put that friendship on a different footing. You are better to find another Reiki Master whose fees you do not mind paying. You will find you enjoy the class more and get along much better with the Reiki Master when you don't have feelings of resentment about fees. Feeling good about the person who teaches you Reiki makes it easy for you to ask questions, learn more and continue the relationship after the class.

I suggest you have some idea why you want to be a Reiki Master. Do you want to do it for your own personal growth or do you want to teach Reiki classes? If you want to do it for personal growth then a Reiki Master who teaches Reiki in a very spiritual way may suit you. If you want to teach Reiki then a Master who includes guidelines and classroom techniques and who shows you how to teach all three levels of Reiki may be better for you. Ask questions. Don't just concentrate on fees, although they can be important because they will determine whether you can or cannot afford the training, other aspects can be just as important. For instance: getting along well with your Reiki Master Teacher, what they teach, when they are able to teach, how long the training will take, and so on.

There is a saying in Reiki that *"you are drawn to the right Reiki Master for you."* Whoever you ultimately choose for your Reiki Master will be the right Reiki Master—regardless of whether you get along with them or not. I have seen this happen over and over again and am amazed at how it works every time. Some people seem to need lessons from a negative perspective and others from a positive one. It will depend on which perspective makes you ask questions and pushes you to practice and strive to learn as much as you can.

DEFINITION OF A REIKI MASTER

The word Master originally was translated from the Japanese word Sensei, which means teacher. The English word 'master' in the 1930s, when Reiki was first translated into English, was commonly used in reference to a teacher. Master also means someone who is very skilled at what they do and a person who has control such as: master of industry, master of the house and master of a college. Therefore some people look at the title of Reiki Master and expect to see someone who is very skilled at Reiki. They also expect someone they can look up to as a leader in the Reiki community.

With Reiki we attend a class, are attuned to that particular class's level of Reiki, given formulas and techniques with which to practice Reiki and then we are left to our own devices to become proficient. This means we can feel like we are only just beginning to be a Master when we have finished our Master class.

3rd Degree Reiki— Master & Teacher

A master is usually someone who has reached a point where they have mastered their training and have enough knowledge and experience to pass it on to others. My experience suggests that the same is true for Reiki. The experience and knowledge you acquire at 1st and 2nd Degree Reiki acts as the foundation of your Reiki Master-ship. The more time you give yourself to become proficient at 1st and 2nd Degree Reiki the more confident you will be in your knowledge and experience of Reiki when you become a Reiki Master.

Master by Example

Regardless of whether you decide to teach Reiki or not, be aware that you and your behavior will be observed by other Reiki Practitioners and by non-Reiki people and compared to your title of Reiki Master. They will look at you as someone skilled and with the ability to be a leader in the Reiki community. Opting out of teaching at Master level does not mean that you are able to also opt out of this aspect of Reiki Master. You will find that if you do not fully step into the role of Reiki Master you will lose the respect of the people around you.

Each degree of Reiki is a new beginning, a new aspect of Reiki. This is especially so when reaching the level of Reiki Master. It expands you and moves you into the unknown parts of your life. The third level of Reiki takes us into the realm beyond the physical and mental/emotional, into the spiritual; that place which belongs to God. This doesn't happen overnight or by the time you have completed your Master training. It evolves gradually as you continue to work with Reiki at the 3rd level.

Your reputation as a Reiki Master will be based on your behavior and your integrity. 'Word of mouth' can travel very quickly within the Reiki community and it doesn't take long for your reputation, either good or bad, to spread. The honesty, principles and morals you bring to your work and your attitudes and actions when you are a Reiki Master will determine the respect that you engender within your students and within the rest of the Reiki community. My advice is to:

- Avoid making any promises you can't keep with grace and goodwill.
- Honor all your commitments.

- Avoid making statements on subjects you don't know or are unsure of.
- If you can't answer a question say so and try to find the answer later.
- Pay your debts.
- Accept that there are differences in how other Reiki Masters teach.
- Avoid boasting about being a Reiki Master and how much energy you access.
- Be aware that excessive pride in being a Reiki Master can be off-putting to others.
- Be kind and considerate to everyone you meet.

Looking After Yourself

Standing in the energy of the 3rd level of Reiki requires you to stay balanced. The energy at Reiki Master level can be exhilarating but you cannot live on it. Your body still requires sleep and food. You can become aware of the Reiki energy the night before a class and you may not feel like sleeping. During a Reiki class the energy may be very noticeable throughout the whole day, not just for the attunement(s), and it will take a while to subside after the class. During this period you may feel you can go without food and sleep.

The feeling of the Reiki energy is wonderful. You will feel elated, on top of the world, but if you don't eat and rest during this period you will find yourself suffering later. Stories abound of Reiki Masters who get ill or burn out soon after becoming Reiki Masters. Learn to honor yourself and your body.

- Try to get to bed at a reasonable hour the night before a class.
- Have something to eat for breakfast—even if it is just toast and tea.
- Drink plenty of water during the class.
- Have a break for something to eat at midday.
- Have an evening meal after the day's class.
- Try to get to bed at a reasonable hour after the class.

Skipping meals is not recommended. Eating a small amount is better than nothing at all. If you feel run-down or tired take vitamins and minerals and do some exercise. Take a serious look at your diet and do some work on improving it. The energy of Reiki activates the body's ability to heal. For the body to heal it needs protein. The more Reiki you do on yourself and others the more likely you are to need a high protein diet. This has meant some people, on reaching Reiki Master level, have changed from being vegetarians to including meat in their diets. Others have found they have increased the amount of fruit and vegetables they eat. Reiki activates the endocrine system to work more efficiently in the body. This system requires vitamins and minerals to work well and many of these can be found in fruit and vegetables although there may be times when you also need to take supplements of vitamins and minerals.

Recommendations

After receiving your Reiki Master attunement do 21 days of self-treatments. If you did not do the 3A/Advanced Reiki Degree then use just the Usui Reiki Master symbol at each hand position so you experience and integrate that symbol on its own. If you have already done a 21 day series of self-treatments using just the Usui Reiki Master symbol then do another 21 days of self-treatments after your Reiki Master attunement using all four Reiki symbols at each hand position.

I also recommend that you practice the attunements you were taught for 1st and 2nd Degree on a doll, teddy bear or pillow until you know the attunement formulas by heart. I suggest you practice until you can do each attunement within 2 minutes. Being able to do an attunement that fast helps you to memorize the attunement and ensures you won't forget it. When you do attunements on your students you will move through the attunement formula at a slower pace as you get into a rhythm with the flow of the energy.

Even if you do not intend to teach Reiki I recommend that you learn the attunements by heart. There may be occasions when you will need to give someone an attunement and it can be embarrassing to say you have forgotten. It also means you will be able to give yourself attunements when you feel the need for them.

If you are a regular member, or the facilitator of, a Reiki Support Group ask the members of the group if you can practice Reiki attunements on them; give 1st Degree practitioners 1st Degree attunements and 2nd Degree practitioners 2nd Degree attunements.

When you give someone an attunement you are also receiving some of that attunement energy. Each attunement you give contributes to your growth on the spiritual level.

REIKI TEACHER

TAKING REIKI INTO THE MARKETPLACE

In my experience teaching Reiki is the biggest learning curve of all the Reiki degrees; sometimes frustrating but always fascinating. I have been fortunate in having students who have not just learned Reiki from me but who have taught me how to improve my life, my teaching methods and who have brought me new ideas, asked questions I have never encountered before, and taught me tolerance and acceptance. Their contributions to my experience as both a Reiki Master and Reiki Teacher have been huge; enabling me to grow, question and search for more understanding about Reiki and people. Teaching students is what makes the Reiki Master level a fascinating experience.

A Reiki Teacher is a Reiki Master who has chosen to teach Reiki to others. You cannot be a Reiki Teacher and not a Reiki Master. To be able to pass on the ability to do Reiki you need to be a Reiki Master.

It is a big step in your Reiki journey to go out and teach Reiki to others, no matter how much training you receive to prepare you for this. Your responsibility as a Master and Teacher is to ensure that all your students leave your class knowing how to use Reiki at the level you have taught them. You are not responsible for making sure they practice after they leave the class but you are responsible for what they learn while they are in your class. Your enthusiasm for Reiki and how you present your classes will encourage students to practice after they leave the class.

Class fees

How much you charge for your Reiki classes is your business and no one else's. What others charge for their classes is their business not yours. You should feel comfortable about what you charge. If you feel undervalued or if you get annoyed because someone else charges more than you then you are probably not charging enough. If you feel guilty about how much you are charging or spend a lot of energy and time explaining why you have chosen your fees then you are probably charging too much. You should feel as comfortable and relaxed about your fees as you do about receiving wages. Try to have as little emotion/attitudes/beliefs etc. attached to your fees as possible. If a student disagrees with how much you charge then suggest they find another Reiki Teacher. Lowering your fees to suit them will create a lack of respect for you and what you teach and they will probably challenge you on other matters to prove they can beat you down on those things as well.

There is nothing to stop you from not charging any fees for Reiki classes except how you feel about it. Remember that the spiritual level is about bringing the physical and mental/emotional worlds or levels together in harmony. If you do not have a deep inner peace about free classes then this can cause your spiritual path to be blocked.

Occasionally a student will ask a Reiki Master if they can pay off their Reiki fees over a period of time. After observing the experiences of quite a number of Reiki Masters it would seem that this option often doesn't work. Some Reiki Masters have had students who did not pay their fees in full. The student soon realizes that a Reiki Master cannot turn off their Reiki if fees are not paid. As a consequence some Reiki Masters do not hand out certificates for Reiki classes until the full fee has been collected and others prefer the fee paid in full before the Master attunement is given. An innovative solution to this problem is for the student to make a series of advance payments to the Reiki Master until the fee is fully paid before the student attends a class.

Certificates

Reiki certificates are a traditional part of the Reiki system. They give the Reiki student pride in having done a Reiki class, a sense of achievement, and a feeling of self-worth. They also indicate that the Reiki Master has a sense of pride in what they are teaching. Your reputation as a Reiki Master and Reiki Teacher can be affected by whether or not you give your students a Reiki Certificate. The most effective advertising for Reiki Masters is 'word of mouth' and complaints spread faster than praise. Your reputation is your responsibility.

One of the most common complaints made about a Reiki Master, which can often hold deep resentment and bitterness, is that the Reiki Master did not give their student(s) a certificate at the end of a Reiki Class and that months or a year or so later, the student still hadn't received a certificate.

A Reiki Certificate can become important for other reasons i.e., as proof that your student has actually attended your Reiki classes. As Reiki becomes more acceptable to mainstream healing the Reiki Certificates also become important should a student apply for a job within a healing establishment as a Reiki Practitioner or when a Reiki Practitioner wants to set up their own healing clinic or if they wish to become a member of a professional body of Natural Health Practitioners.

Check Lists

There are everyday bits and pieces that need to be done to ensure your classes run smoothly. Using a 'check list' that lists all the equipment you need and all the steps to take i.e., advertising, receipts, certificates, etc., can ensure you don't miss something.

Date of the Class

This will be set by either yourself or by mutual agreement with your student or students. Once you have set a date it is advisable to keep to that date. People do not like Masters who regularly cancel classes or change dates —students have their own plans and are busy people too.
   a. Ensure that you have a venue available to use on that day.
   b. Advertise your class.
   c. Do the energy work for your class (send absent healing to ensure your class is a success).
   d. When you know who your students will be prepare certificates, manuals, receipts, etc.

Duration of the Class

Decide how long your class is going to take. Not everyone has their own transport so some students like to know when the class will finish so that they can arrange for someone to take them home. Other members of your class may have plans for activities after the class that they need to be on time to attend. Once you have decided on your class program it is a good idea to take one or two friends or relatives for the first class or do a dress rehearsal of your class using dolls or soft toys as your students.

The duration of your class will depend on the format of your class, the information you intend to pass on to the student, how much practice you get the students to do, how much time you allow for breaks and for questions and answers. The number of people you have in a class and how many attunements you give them will need to be factored into the class timeframe.

Venue

If you are going to teach classes at home ensure you won't be disturbed by family members, other people living in the house, or by visitors. Your home should be clean and tidy as it will act as a symbol and example of you and your Reiki Master-ship.

If you have the use of a friend's or student's home, find out what the friend or student expects from you. For example, what time they would like the class to start and finish, use of other parts of the house such as kitchen, toilet and bathroom, what happens if there are any breakages, who provides lunch and so on. It is better to sort things out prior to a class so there are no misconceptions and misunderstandings. That way you will be welcome to teach there again.

If you rent a venue don't forget to ask for the latest cancellation date should you not get any students. Not notifying the venue owner within an agreed-upon timeframe that you have cancelled a class can result in you being liable for the full rental of the venue.

It is preferable to rent a venue you are familiar with as this will help you maintain your self-confidence. If you haven't seen the venue before, try to visit it prior to the class or go to the venue earlier than you usually would before the start of a class. Find out:
  a. where the toilets are and whether you need to supply towels, toilet paper and soap.
  b. what is available in the kitchen such as plates, cups, cutlery, towels, detergent, etc.
  c. how many chairs are available.
  d. whether there is enough room to put up massage tables.
  e. how you are going to set out the room for your class.
  f. if there is a heating system and how to use it.

Not all venues are kept clean and at some places I have had to vacuum, sweep, wipe down benches, clean toilets and clear away lingering smells before a class. Venues usually have the cleaning materials, but I take dusters, liquid bleach (cleans toilets quickly), cleansers and detergent with me when I rent a venue. I have found perfumed candles and incense help to clear musty and nasty smells from a room or rooms. Regardless of how you have found a venue it is recommended you leave it clean and tidy at the end of the day. Usually your students will happily help you clear up without being asked.

Advertising

Once you have decided on how long your class will be and when and where you are going to hold it, you can then advertise. There are a variety of ways to advertise your class. The Internet allows you to put in place advertising that is constantly available to Internet browsers and it is a good place for cheap, long term advertising. Many local high schools hold night classes where you can learn to write your own web page. Small regular advertisements in your local newspaper or natural health magazines are a good option but can be costly. You can also send out regular newsletters to your students, or you can rely on 'word of mouth'. Libraries, health food shops, supermarkets and community centers have message boards for local advertising. You may need to get approval before placing your advertisement on their board.

Preparing for the Class

To save time and prevent a last minute rush, prepare certificates, receipts and any written material such as manuals or notes prior to the class.

You can also send Reiki via Distance/Absent Healing to the time and place of your Reiki classes. This ensures everything will go well for the highest good of all concerned. You can also send Reiki to attract students to your class. You can send out an intent for the number of people you would like to attend your class but you will soon learn that Reiki does not manipulate people into your class. You will get the numbers and people who are right for you and your class and that may be less or more than you asked for. Sending energy, I have found, seems to bring everything together smoothly. If, for any reason, you have chosen the wrong day or venue, information will be forthcoming that will allow you to make necessary changes with the least amount of fuss.

3rd Degree Reiki— Master & Teacher

Prior to Arrival

Be ready for your class well before your students arrive. Give yourself time to set up your room (if you haven't done so the evening before) and ensure you have plenty of water and glasses available. Take some time to sit quietly in the room. Use Reiki and the Reiki symbols to center yourself and prepare for the class. This allows you to be relaxed and ready for your students and enables you to handle whatever happens during the day. Use the Reiki symbols to clear, cleanse and bless the room so that the atmosphere feels welcoming and is conducive to learning.

On Arrival

By the time your students begin arriving you should be physically, mentally and emotionally ready for them. Greet each person as they arrive, introduce yourself, find out who they are, accept their payment for the class and give them a receipt. Show them where they can put their coats and bags, where they can find the toilet, and where the class will be held.

Start the Class

Ensure the class starts on time. At this point put the money you have received for the class away both physically and mentally. Forget any personal problems. Don't worry about whether you have forgotten to do something. If you have, deal with it when required. Go into your class with your focus on teaching Reiki to your students.

Close the Class

At the end of the class:

a. Hand out Reiki certificates (if you don't have them ready, ensure you send them out within the first two weeks after the class, which is the grace period most people mentally allow for something to be sent to them).

b. Hand out any pamphlets, manuals, and other information you would like your students to take away with them.

c. If you wish, give everyone a hug (if you are the hugging kind). Although hugging is endemic within the Reiki community, it is not compulsory and if you don't feel comfortable about hugging you don't have to.

d. Make sure no one has left anything behind.

e. Clean and tidy the venue. Pack up all your equipment. Ensure you haven't left anything behind. If students offer to help you, accept with grace and thanks.

GENERAL REMARKS ABOUT TEACHING

If you are unsure about teaching attend a class that teaches you how to teach adults. In New Zealand these classes are held at Polytechnics—technical colleges that are an alternative to universities. These classes are usually taught to people who want to teach night classes at High Schools, or for work-place educators as well as for the many people who teach self-help and metaphysical classes.

Effective learning takes place when a number of the senses are used. Reiki Masters generally use three of the senses to teach Reiki—sound, sight and touch.

a.	Sound	Explain
b.	Sight	Demonstrate
c.	Touch	Practice

Try to incorporate these three aspects into your class as much as possible. You can also include emotion by bringing in a sense of humor and by expressing your enthusiasm for Reiki during the class.

By Example

Be aware that you will also be teaching by example. This can be either a negative or a positive example. The example you present as a Reiki Master will depend on the impressions, judgments and expectations of your students, friends and family.

Many of the impressions that your students get about you will be formed by how you teach the class and interact with them, not from what you teach. The impact you make on your students (and other people you mix with at work and socially) will have an impact on your reputation as a Reiki Master. Impressions tend to be tied up with feelings; how comfortable or uncomfortable a person feels when they are with you.

Children learn by copying what the people around them say and do. We do not lose this ability when we become adults. It is something that remains with us all our lives. By adulthood we have also learned to make judgments about people. The judgments made by your students will also impact on your reputation as a Reiki Master. Sometimes these judgments can seem unfair. As a Reiki Master you need to be aware that you can control these judgments by your behavior and the example you set. Use such judgments to teach you to improve your presentation of Reiki and to improve yourself.

Many people have an expectation of what a Reiki Master is like before actually meeting one. They may have expectations of perfection, good health, success, kindness and other such qualities. The more praise someone has heard about a Reiki Master the greater the expectation.

No-one is perfect, and that includes Reiki Masters. I believe a Reiki Master's journey is to move towards bringing all aspects of yourself together, to express the whole of yourself, and to live in balance and harmony with yourself and in compassion with others. This is a life-long journey that requires you to be aware of what is positive and negative in your life. For instance, a sarcastic sense of humor can be amusing at times but it can also be hurtful and holds little or no compassion for others. Cultivate a sense of humor that contains kindness. Develop the qualities of patience, tolerance and acceptance for they help you to deal with the variety of people who come to your classes.

Teaching Style

How you teach a Reiki class will depend on how you learned each of your Reiki degrees, how you were taught to teach Reiki when you were training to be a Reiki Master and your own opinions and experience of Reiki.

Each student is drawn to the right Reiki Master. It will be your personality, how you conduct yourself as a Reiki Master and the way you teach that will draw students to you. The Laws of Attraction include 'like attracting like' and also the attraction of opposites. Students will be drawn to you because they have a personality that is similar or like your own or opposite to yours. The students whose personalities are opposite to yours will often be the hardest to teach but they will be the ones who will teach you how to be a better teacher if you are willing to recognize the lessons.

You will have people in your class who are outgoing and extroverted and others who are shy, some who are happy, some who are unhappy and others who live their lives somewhere in between. Some students will be talkative and others quiet, some will be independent and others will want to be dependent. Each will challenge you in some way. Just when you think you are able to cope with all types of people someone will turn up who is aggressive and challenges everything you say and do, thereby making you aware of how little you know, how you feel when your authority as a teacher is challenged, what you value and how to maintain your own values. Then you may encounter the needy who want all of your attention and the attention of the rest of your class. They will sabotage your time and drain your energy. From them you will learn to keep your class running on schedule, how to remain energized, and how to be compassionate yet detached.

Your teaching style will evolve as you evolve as a Reiki Master. Your confidence and ability to impart information to students will improve. The more classes you teach the more proficient you will become.

In the Class

Keep your attention on your class and their needs. Don't become distracted or allow your mind to wander. If your thoughts and energies are focused on your own personal problems you will not be able to do a good job of teaching your class and you will offend or hurt someone by your lack of attention and focus.

Keep to the subject of Reiki. If someone begins to talk about their personal problems, family, etc. gently bring the subject back to Reiki. Don't talk about your problems, family, etc. unless it is to specifically illustrate a point about how Reiki helped you to overcome a problem.

Keep your personal Reiki stories brief. By all means answer questions about Reiki or illustrate a point with a personal experience, but don't waffle on and on. You have a lot to teach in the class and cannot afford to spend too much time on long meandering explanations.

Always remain aware of your students and what they are doing. Take notice of whether they understand what you are teaching them. Give them time to ask questions if they are not sure about something. Check that they understand, can follow and practice the lessons as you have demonstrated.

Answer questions. You will probably be able to answer most of the questions your students are likely to ask from your own personal experience, from what you have been taught about Reiki, and from what you have read. If you are not able to answer a question, tell the student that you have not had that experience with Reiki so cannot give them an answer. Point out that Reiki always works for the highest good and can do no harm and that perhaps they should try using Reiki themselves for the situation they are asking about to find out what will happen.

Encourage your students to talk in the class. Allow time for people to talk about what they are experiencing. This can be done by asking each person to explain how they felt and what they experienced during an attunement or treatment and after they have done a particular exercise in the class such as absent healing, using the symbols, etc. This can lead to the student or students feeling relaxed and confident about asking questions. It also helps the student to become more observant of the shifts and changes that take place in their life and the areas where they have pain, are not happy or perhaps need to work on for healing to occur.

Make no judgments about your students. You are teaching them Reiki because they have been drawn to your expression of the universal life force energy. At the same time you have been drawn to their energy. Remember the best teachers learn from their students. If a student or students push your buttons and upset you during a class, this is an area you need to look at for your own health and well being. Take time out after the class to reflect on why you became upset. Don't blame the student. Often they don't realize they have upset you or why. When you become upset it is your button and your problem that has been activated not theirs. You need to take time in the days after the class to recognize why you became upset and to send Reiki to the problem so that it can be healed.

Class Plan

I have found that writing a class plan of what I intend to teach is a good idea. It enables me to focus on what I want to do in my class. It also provides me with guidelines that keep me from being sidetracked and helps me to stay aware of the time.

NOTES ON TEACHING 1ST DEGREE REIKI

Setting Up the Venue for 1st Degree

How you arrange the set up of your venue for 1st Degree will depend on the space you have available. It is a good idea, if possible, to have sufficient space for your students to move around the venue (have a change of scene). In a large room you may be able to set up four separate areas:

1. an area where students sit to hear history, terminology, do a self-treatment and a chair treatment.
2. an area where attunements take place.
3. an area with massage tables set up (do this before the start of class if possible).
4. an area for lunch and morning/afternoon breaks.

If the area is small you may have to move chairs away to put up massage tables and hold attunements in another room.

Seated Area—This can be a circle of chairs or pillows. Make sure this area is reasonably comfortable because your students will be using this area for quite a while.

Attunement Area—How you lay out your attunement area is entirely up to you and will be influenced by the space that is available and the way you prefer doing attunements. I like doing my attunements in a circle with the students facing the center. If the area is large enough, I decorate the center of the circle with flowers and a candle.

Treatment Area—Have enough space around the massage table or tables for practitioners to walk down at least one side of the table and to have a chair placed at each end of the table. There should be enough space for the practitioner to be comfortable when he/she gives a Reiki treatment.

What to teach in a 1st Degree class

The basic subjects taught at 1st Degree are: the history, information about Reiki, hand positions for a self-treatment, and hand positions for treating other people. How you teach 1st Degree Reiki will depend on how you learned the degree yourself, how you were taught to teach it and how you would personally like to teach it.

3rd Degree Reiki—Master & Teacher

History

The history of Reiki has changed since additional information was discovered about Mikao Usui. The original 'Reiki Story' about Mikao Usui's journey up the mountain is now recognized as a mythical story—not factual but still containing 'truths' about Reiki. The Reiki history can be divided into two parts—the biographical information about the founder, Mikao Usui, and those who brought Reiki to the West and the mythical story of Reiki. As the teacher it is your choice how you present these two strands of information.

Today, when teaching the history of Reiki, you have the choice of telling the Reiki Story as Mrs. Takata told it or just using the biographical stories of Mikao Usui, Chijuro Hayashi and Mrs. Hawayo Takata, or including both the mythical Reiki Story and the biographical history in your class. I like to start the History by telling my students the biological facts about Mikao Usui, Chijuro Hayashi and then Mrs. Takata. Then I move into the Reiki Story by saying that this was the way Mrs. Takata told it when she first brought Reiki to the West. During the story I point out various places within the story that show you how to use Reiki.

The Biographical History

How you want to present this information is entirely up to you. Details about Mikao Usui are to be found in the books by Frank Arjava Petter. The details about Chujiro Hayashi and Mrs. Hawayo Takata are to be found in the stories about Mrs. Takata. I suggest the biographical history can include:

a. When and where Mikao Usui was born.
b. Going to Kurama where he experienced Reiki.
c. Mikao Usui's tombstone—where it is, its inscription and what to do when you visit it.
d. Chijuro Hayashi and his clinic in Tokyo.
e. Mrs. Takata being born in Hawaii and her visit to Japan.
f. Mrs. Takata being healed at Chijuro Hayashi's clinic.
g. Mrs. Takata becomes a Reiki Practitioner and works in Hayashi's clinic.
h. Mrs. Takata brings Reiki to the West.

The Mythical Reiki Story

When telling the mythical Reiki Story it is acceptable to read it aloud in your class like a story. This should be done in a believable way. I think the story should contain the following elements:

a. Mikao Usui's search for a natural method of healing.

b. His arrival and study at the Zen Monastery in Kyoto.

c. Finding the method but not the power to heal.

d. His visit to the sacred mountain, Kurama, outside Kyoto to meditate and fast.

e. Being hit by the light and learning from the colored bubbles of light.

f. The healing he did on his way back to the monastery:

    i. Healing his stubbed toe (indicates Reiki heals injuries/surgery).

    ii. Healing the girl with a toothache (indicates permission needs to be given when a client or yourself has a list of reasons why they can't be healed).

    iii. Eating a large meal after fasting.

g. Arriving back at the monastery:

    i. Changing clothes and bathing.

    ii. Healing the abbot's arthritis.

h. Going to the Beggar City in Kyoto (that part of us that has a poverty mentality).

i. Discovering that the beggars had not changed their lives.

j. Returning to the monastery to meditate on how to improve Reiki.

    i. Five Reiki Principles (explain these).

    ii. Energy Exchange (explain this).

    iii. Not forcing Reiki on anyone (explain this).

k. Traveling around Japan—standing in the marketplace with a torch.

Terminology and Ideology

Like every other modality Reiki has certain terms that are used by Reiki Practitioners that may not be known to others. For example: Master/Sensei, Reiki, shifts, healing crisis, etc. Also, some of your students may not have had much to do with ideas such as the universal life force energy, energy being moved by intent, and energy having its own knowingness or intelligence. Some people are not aware that many illnesses have an emotional/psychological cause or background. You need to spend some time explaining these terms and ideas. Most of your students' questions will probably be about these aspects of Reiki.

Hand Positions

You need to show your students how to give themselves a self-treatment and how to treat someone else. I like to show my students at least two ways to treat someone—in a chair and on a table.

Explain   How and where to place their hands, then

Demonstrate   Show them how and where to place their hands, then

Practice   Get them to place their hands in the positions described, by allowing them to:

   a. do a self-treatment.

   b. give a treatment to a student who is sitting in a chair.

   c. give a treatment to a student lying on a table.

Although Reiki can be used intuitively, the traditional twelve hand positions are a good basic starting place for students. They enable students to have the confidence to offer Reiki treatments to other people soon after doing 1st Degree Reiki. As they practice Reiki they will gain confidence and experience in using Reiki intuitively.

Attunement at 1st Degree

Mrs. Takata gave four attunements to each of her students during a 1st Degree class. Three of the attunements were said to be temporary and that if a student left a Reiki class before receiving the fourth attunement their connection with Reiki would fade away after a few weeks. My initial understanding of these four attunements is that they enabled students to practice Reiki in the class before having to confirm they wanted to be connected to Reiki for the rest of their lives. Consequently many lineages of Reiki today only do the permanent Reiki attunement during a 1st Degree class. I was taught to do just one attunement but found that I felt uncomfortable about that and for a while gave my students two permanent attunements—one at the beginning of the class and the second at the end of the class. Eventually I decided to give my students four attunements (all permanent) during a 1st Degree class and found I felt much more satisfied with that number of attunements for 1st Degree.

The number of attunements you give during a 1st Degree class will be influenced by the number given by the Master who trained you to be a Reiki Master. If you don't feel happy about just doing one attunement there is room to experiment.

If you choose to give more than one attunement at 1st Degree it is best if your students receive a Reiki treatment between each attunement. This helps them to assimilate and integrate the attunement. For example, 1st attunement followed by a self-treatment, 2nd attunement followed by a treatment while sitting in a chair, 3rd attunement followed by a treatment while lying on a massage table, and the 4th attunement prior to leaving the class to be followed by the students doing 21 days of self-treatments on themselves after the class.

The comments about Temporary Heart Attunements in this book in the section on 3A/Advance Reiki Degree also apply to giving attunements for the 1st, 2nd, and 3rd Degrees.

Results

Your students should leave your class confident about giving themselves and others Reiki treatments. They should also feel confident enough to join a Reiki Support Group in their local area. Support Groups enable students to practice Reiki, receive Reiki and have a place where they can ask questions and share their experiences of using Reiki. Another gift you can give to your students is enthusiasm for Reiki. That enthusiasm will ensure they keep practicing Reiki on themselves. If you express your own enthusiasm for Reiki openly and honestly it will be contagious. Answering questions honestly will also help your students to trust the process of Reiki and help them to continue practicing.

NOTES ON TEACHING 2ND DEGREE REIKI

Setting Up A Venue for 2nd Degree

A 2nd Degree Reiki class is more simple to set up. You will need a place for your student/students to sit, to write, to practice the symbols and to have an attunement. Conducting a full Reiki treatment on a table is optional during a 2nd Degree class. Instead you can give a short demonstration of how to use the Reiki symbols during a treatment. The students can then practice on themselves by doing a self-treatment chakra balance or by giving each other a short treatment while sitting in a chair. If you do want your 2nd Degree students to give each other Reiki treatments on massage tables, your venue needs to be big enough to set up the required number of tables.

What to Teach at 2nd Degree

There are three basic subjects taught at 2nd Degree Reiki.
1. The first three Reiki symbols.
2. Mental/Emotional hand position.
3. Distance/Absent Healing.

As Reiki has passed down through the lineages from Mrs. Takata 2nd Degree Reiki has changed—symbols have altered and there are now a variety of ways to do Distance/Absent Healing. There is often a lot more information included at 2nd Degree than was originally taught because successive Masters have also included their experiences of using the Reiki symbols into this degree. You will probably do the same.

The main objective of 2nd Degree is to teach the first three Reiki symbols and to ensure that your students know and understand how to use them. A large portion of your class time will be spent teaching people how to say and draw the three symbols. Although people seem to have a greater concept of symbols today than they did a few years ago there is still a need to explain, at least briefly, what symbols are and how they work.

When it comes to teaching 2nd Degree Reiki, I believe, you need to be confident and experienced in using the Reiki symbols. Learn as much as you can about the 2nd Degree symbols. The more you use the symbols on yourself and understand them the easier it is to introduce them to others. This is achieved by using the symbols every day, trying out new ideas and ways of using them, and being aware of what happens to you, to your environment and to others when you use them. For me the symbols are three-dimensional living beings who live on the invisible plane and who are happy to assist us on this plane. They are my best friends and I feel sad whenever I hear someone say they are just something on which to focus the mind, or that we don't need them.

Some Masters include a number of other subjects in their 2nd Degree class such as chakras and chakra balancing, other symbols, crystals, divination cards, other modalities, etc. What you include in your class will depend on the amount of time you have available after teaching the three basic subjects of 2nd Degree Reiki. The range of subjects and the time spent on each subject will determine the length of your class i.e., one day, two half days, two full days, three evenings, etc. I prefer to keep to the subject of Reiki during Reiki classes and to set up separate classes for other subjects.

The Symbols

The 2nd Degree Reiki symbols are usually taught in the following order:

1st Symbol	Power Symbol	Physical level of 2nd Degree
2nd Symbol	Mental/Emotional Symbol	Mental/Emotional level of 2nd Degree
3rd Symbol	Distance Symbol	Spiritual level of 2nd Degree

Each degree of Reiki contains within it aspects of the three levels; physical (outer world), mental/emotional (inner world), and spiritual (intangible world). In 2nd Degree Reiki these levels are found within the three symbols. As you teach these symbols in the above order you are symbolically moving the student through these three levels, allowing them to realize that they can cope with the increasing difficulties of each level. Each symbol becomes more intricate, moving from the simple spiral of the Power Symbol to the five overlapping Kanji characters of the Distance Symbol. By starting with the simple Power Symbol you also do not overwhelm the student who may never have worked with symbols before.

Students require time to practice drawing the symbols and you need to pay attention to what they are doing. I try to ensure that my students draw each of the symbols at least 15 times on paper; because I was once told that writing something 15 times or more will take the information past the ego and into the subconscious mind. I then instruct them to practice drawing the symbols in the air with their hands, using first their fingertips and then the center of their palm. Once they are comfortable with that I instruct them to draw the symbols with their mind's eye.

1. Ask the student(s) to close their eyes (it is easier for a beginner to draw the symbols with their eyes closed). Having their eyes closed

also means they do not move their physical eyes while mentally drawing the symbols.

2. Ask them to focus on their inner sight just above their eyes in the center of their forehead—which is approximately where their third eye resides.
3. Instruct them to imagine a beam of light coming out of their third eye.
4. Next, ask them to draw the symbol with the beam of light. I tell them to try to move the beam not to their heads while they are drawing symbols.
5. Tell them to think of the name of the symbol three times either while drawing the symbol or after they have completed it.

The Mental/Emotional Technique

This technique is traditionally taught at 2nd Degree level because it involves the use of the first two Reiki symbols. Explain the steps as you demonstrate this technique on a student sitting in a chair.

1. Place one hand on the head, either on the forehead or back of the head.
2. Draw the Mental/Emotional symbol over the top of the head. Show your students that you draw the symbol in the air, without touching the hair so the receiver doesn't feel what is happening.
3. The next step is to press the symbol gently into the receiver's head as you think the name of the symbol three times. Advise your students not to press too hard.
4. Then do the same for the Power Symbol.
5. Finally place the hand you drew the symbols with on the back of the head, or on the forehead opposite your other hand, or on the top of the head. Tell your students that they can hold this position from six minutes or more. The longer this position can be held the better.
6. Get your students to give each other the mental/emotional technique for at least 6 minutes. If you have only one student, give him/her the technique and then get him/her to give you one.

Distance/Absent Healing

The basic Distance/Absent Healing technique is:

a. Draw the Distance Symbol.
b. Say the name of the symbol three times.

c. Say the name of the person or event three times.

d. Place your hands on a witness/proxy/surrogate (yourself/paper/doll, etc).

Some Reiki students are taught to begin their Distance/Absent Healing with the Power and Mental/Emotional symbols to clear themselves first before sending. Personally, I find the Dry Bathing technique is a really effective method for clearing myself before doing Distance/Absent Healing and also to disconnect afterwards.

There are numerous witnesses you can use for Distance/Absent Healing. I suggest that you don't overwhelm your students by trying to include all of them in your class. Give them enough to ensure that they know they can be flexible and so they realize there is not just one 'right' way of doing Distance Healing. Some of the ways of 'witnessing' during Distance/Absent Healing are:

1. Write name(s) of person/people on paper and hold the paper between your hands.
2. Write an event for the past or future on paper and hold the paper between your hands.
3. Place your hands on a photograph of a person or a group of people.
4. Do all the Reiki hand positions on a pillow or doll/teddy bear.
5. Use the standard Reiki hand positions for Distance/Absent Healing—which is to place hands on knees/thighs.
6. Finger technique—joining thumb and index finger together to make a circle.
7. Place your hands on your solar plexus or heart chakra.
8. Cup your hands together and visualize the person between them.
9. Mentally invite the person to stand before you and visualize them there. Hold your palms towards them and beam Reiki at them.

Give your students time to practice sending Distance/Absent Healing using several different witnesses. For example:

1. Send to one person—a friend or relative using a photograph and/or a pillow or by half your class sending to the other half.
2. Send to a group of people whose names are listed on a piece of paper.

3. Write a future event on a piece of paper and send Reiki to it i.e., birthday, wedding, family event, job interview, purchase of a new house or car, exam, first date, etc.
4. Place hands on the solar plexus and send to an event in the past— 1st day at school, an accident, first 7 years of life, a stay in the hospital, a broken relationship, etc.
5. Send to a past life using the finger technique of forming a circle with thumb and index finger.

After each experience allow each student to talk about it. If they are not sure what to say prompt them by asking what happened and how they felt about it. However, if the experience has been very personal and private don't push the student to reveal all; allow them their privacy.

Other Ways of Using the Symbols

There are many ways of using the Reiki symbols. By teaching those that you have used and experienced you will have more credibility and confidence during the class. Here are a few ways of explaining and/or demonstrating the use of symbols:
1. Demonstrate, then get students to draw a large symbol, and step into it. They should start drawing the symbol in the air above their heads and finish the symbol at their feet. Having their eyes closed while they stand in the symbol will open their inner senses to the energy of the symbol. When they step out of the symbol ask each person how they felt and what they experienced. Get them to do this with all three symbols.
2. Demonstrate placing the symbols in a doorway. Draw the symbols from the top of the doorway down to the floor.
3. Demonstrate placing the symbols on a bed (use a chair or sofa to demonstrate on). You can ask your students to stand up and place the symbols into the chair they have been sitting on.
4. Explain how to place the symbols on cars, houses, boats, luggage and other possessions, and why they would want to do this.
5. If you have time, get your students to give each other a Reiki treatment using all three symbols. They can do this as a full treatment on a massage table, or sitting in a chair, or as a self-treatment. Ask your students to:
   a. draw the Power symbol on their hands before starting the treat-

ment to activate the flow of more energy.

b. draw the three symbols at each hand position of the treatment.

c. intuitively choose a specific area of the body then draw the Power Symbol in their mouth and blow it over the chosen spot.

d. ask their intuition how many Power symbols (or other symbols) are needed to cleanse the receiver's lungs. Then do it again for the liver and kidneys.

e. finish the treatment by mentally drawing the Distance Symbol down the back of the receiver.

6. When you take a meal or break get the students to bless their food/water/tea by drawing the Power Symbol over it.

7. Demonstrate how to clear the energy in a room and use the symbols to activate the room's Feng Shui by drawing the symbols in each of the corners and in the center of the room.

8. Get your students to refresh their facial muscles by drawing the Power Symbol on their fingers and hands before stroking their face.

9. At the end of the class guide your students through the Pink Happiness Power Symbol.

Chakra Balance

The idea of chakras and balancing the chakras is often introduced at 2nd Degree Reiki level. The chakra system is an Eastern understanding of the major energy system of the body. It corresponds to the endocrine system that is the Western understanding of the body's major energy system. Explaining the chakra system is easier than explaining the more technical endocrine system. As information about alternative ways of healing has become more widespread many students will already have heard of the chakra system.

Taking students through a Chakra Balance Self-treatment is a way of getting them to practice the symbols and their names as well as helping them to integrate their 2nd Degree attunement. It is another way of doing a Reiki treatment. You can write a guided meditation for a Chakra Balance Self-Treatment that you can read aloud to your students. Include in the meditation the names and colors of the chakras, what each chakra represents, when to change hand positions and when to draw a symbol, what symbol to draw and how to visualize it going into a chakra.

The 2nd Degree Attunement

There are a number of ways of doing the 2nd Degree attunement among the different lineages of Reiki. Some Reiki Masters give a separate attunement for each symbol and other Reiki Masters attune only the dominant hand with the symbols. My preference is to attune both hands with the symbols during one attunement. My observation is that each version of the attunement works and there seems to be no real difference between them. My thought about attuning only the dominant hand is that there may be times when you may need to use the non-dominant hand to activate the symbols. The major difference I have noted is that when the Power Symbol is activated in a 1st Degree attunement and not during the 2nd Degree attunement it doesn't work as described for the second level of Reiki. If you want it to work as an activating energy and a royal command then it needs to be activated during the 2nd Degree attunement.

TEACHING CHILDREN

I have to admit to never having held a Reiki class for children. The main reason is that I am too serious and do not have a "fun" approach when I am with children. I believe that to teach children well you need to approach the class with fun, happiness and light-heartedness and have easy access to your own "Inner Child". However, after saying that, I would like to offer some suggestions about teaching children Reiki.

Permission

You should always get permission from one or both parents before attuning a child to Reiki. This is for your own benefit. You could find yourself in legal trouble if you interfere with the beliefs and wishes of parents. Many Reiki Masters will not attune a child unless one or both parents are Reiki Practitioners so the child has access to someone with a knowledge and understanding of Reiki and can help the child practice Reiki and also talk about Reiki with them. Some Reiki Masters like a parent to accompany their child to the Reiki class.

It is probably a good idea not to train a child any higher than 1st Degree Reiki. Once the child has reached 16 years or more he/she can make up his/her own mind about whether they want to carry on to 2nd Degree or not. Under 16 years of age they will be strongly influenced by their parents so a decision to take a Reiki course may not necessarily be completely their own.

One-to-One

I have attuned very ill children to Reiki. I give them the 1st Degree attunement (one attunement method) and spend time telling them that whenever they feel tired, in pain or sick they should put their hands on themselves and know that Reiki is helping them. I have never charged for doing this. I have always had the consent of the child's guardian before doing the attunement. I also point out to the parent(s) that Reiki may not save their child's life, but it will help relieve pain and assist them through whatever process is right for them.

Classes for Children

I would include children from 11 years of age in an adult class. They should be able to cope with being part of an adult class. Otherwise teach a separate class for 11 to 16 year olds

Remember that children have a shorter attention span than adults and it is harder to get the whole class to all pay attention at the same time—unless you are a very experienced teacher. By keeping each part of your class short, fun and interesting you should retain the focus of your students. You can also arrange for some of the parents to attend the class so they can help you manage the children.

You will need to determine how much you charge children—many Masters charge half price for under 16 years olds.

The Reiki Story and Principles

I believe the Reiki Story (although not true) is an important aspect of Reiki providing archetypes that work deeply in the mental/emotional and spiritual levels of a person's being. Children enjoy a good story when it is read well. They will not mind if you read it aloud from a book. At the end of the story ask them questions about what they heard and discuss their ideas about what they think of the story.

Don't forget to include an explanation of the Reiki Principles in your class. Discuss with the children what they think about the principles; what they do and don't like about them and what the principles mean.

Attuning Children

Small children are likely to become restless sitting in an attunement circle so it is probably better to attune them one at a time. You may choose to give them one sealed 1st Degree Attunement or all four First Degree attunements.

Don't take too long doing the attunement. Older children won't mind how long you take but younger ones can get restless. During his attunement my four year old nephew opened one eye just as I was about to blow on his hands and asked, "How much longer are you going to be, Aunty Maureen?" I almost choked as I tried to blow and not laugh at the same time.

Having a parent or parents attending the class will ensure the children are supervised while you are doing attunements. Give the children who are waiting or have received their attunement some paper and lots of colored felt tip pens and get them to draw the following:
1. place one of their hands on a piece of paper and trace around it.
2. draw a happy smiling face in the middle of the hand they have traced.
3. draw lines radiating out from the hand and fingers (like they do when they draw sunbeams) to show the energy flow coming from the hand.
4. then do the same with their other hand.
5. draw all the things they can give Reiki to—Mom and Dad, brothers and sisters, cats, dogs, plants, knees, feet, eyes and so on.

A Reiki Song

If you like music you can teach the children the following song about Reiki or make up one of your own.

Magic Hands *(sung to the tune of "Campdown Races")*
Reiki hands are magic hands, do da, do da
Reiki hands are happy hands, all the live long day
They can heal cuts
They can heal bumps
They can make you smile again, all the live long day.
(Repeat)

Self-treatment

Show the children how to do a Reiki self-treatment. Go over the hand positions several times. You can get them to chant or sing the following (or make up your own chant) with you:

Number One is over my eyes to make them sparkle,
Number Two is over my ears to help me hear,
Number Three's the back of my head so I remember well,
Number Four is around my throat to help me say what I mean,
and Number Five is over my heart for lots and lots of love.
Number Six, over my middle helps to build my confidence,
Number Seven is on my tummy so I can feel calm,
Number Eight's where my legs join my body and help me move and
    run around.
Number Nine is over my shoulders to relax.
Number Ten, one on my heart and one on my back then change
    around.
Number Eleven is on my back below my waist where I bend
and last of all is Number Twelve with both hands on the bone where
    a tail could be.

Treating Others

Children are often on the scene first when there is an accident at home, in the playground, at school and other areas where children get together. I believe the emphasis, when it comes to children treating others, should be on what to do at an accident. Get them to pretend they are at an accident—let them all take a turn at being the victim, the Reiki person and the person who goes for help.

At an accident—with other children to help:

1. Stay calm—place your hands on your tummy if you feel afraid.
2. Get someone to go and get help from an adult or phone the emergency number—in some countries this is 911 and in other countries it is 111. Have a discussion about the number.
3. Only move the injured person if it is dangerous to leave them where they are. Discuss what would be a dangerous situation, when you would have to move someone away from the situation (because they may be burned, drowned or hit by something), and when it

would be dangerous to touch an injured person (because of electrical wires).

4. If it is not dangerous, place your hands on the person who is hurt—do not touch the injury.
5 Tell the injured person they will be okay and someone has gone for help.
7. Keep giving them Reiki until an adult comes to help.

At an accident—with only you and the person hurt:
1. Stay calm—place your hands on your tummy.
2. Don't move the person who is hurt unless it is dangerous to leave them there.
3. Make sure they are warm.
4. Phone the emergency number or go get help from an adult.
5. Return and give the injured person Reiki until help arrives.

Full Reiki Treatment

Instruct the children where to place their hands during a Reiki treatment. Have them give each other a Reiki treatment. Tell them when to change positions and tell them where to put their hands next. Give them about one to two minutes in each hand position. Children can get restless and may not be able to give a full hour's treatment—most children (having a smaller body mass) don't always need a full hour's treatment.

NOTES ON TEACHING REIKI WITH CRYSTALS

Students in this class do not receive an attunement/initiation, therefore it can be taught by someone who isn't a Reiki Teacher. For example, students can learn about using Reiki with Crystals by reading through the notes in this book. Many people prefer to learn about using Reiki from a Reiki Teacher. To teach this class you need to have practiced using crystals with Reiki yourself. I recommend that you also read several books about crystals so that you are familiar with their metaphysical qualities and the various ways other people use them.

I try to make this class as much fun as possible. I discovered that it is best to have sets of crystals to use in the class. Some people will bring along crystals when asked, others forget, and others will bring along crystals that are too big and heavy to use in a treatment. I have six sets of quartz crystals (a set includes one each of rose quartz, tourmalated quartz, rutilated quartz, amethyst, smokey quartz and four clear quartz). I also have three sets of the family of chalcedony (one each of rose quartz, citron chrysophase and blood-stone; two chalcedony; and four red jasper). These are the stones that my students practice treatments with. These stones belong to me and I keep them so I can use them in my next class. After each class I soak the stones in salted water then store each set in their own calico bag until the next class or next time they are needed.

At the beginning of the class I lay out a variety of small crystals that can be held comfortably in the hand, about 30-50, on a small table and ask my students to choose eight of them each. They use these crystals they have chosen to practice programming, channeling and distance/absent healing. They take these crystals home with them so they have them to practice with until they are able to buy further crystals themselves. I then hand out my manual about using Reiki with Crystals (which appears as the chapter on Reiki and Crystals in this book) and we go through it step by step.

The steps I take my students through are:
1. Explain what crystals are and do and how to clean and energize them with Reiki.
2. Get the students to intuitively choose 8 crystals for themselves.
3. Get the students to program their chosen crystals with Reiki.
4. Get them to choose four Angel Cards and program their qualities into four of their crystals.
5. Get the students to program Happiness into one of their crystals.
6. Get the students to use a quartz crystal to channel the energy of another crystal.
7. Get the students to give each other a Reiki and Crystal treatment.
8. Do Distance/Absent Healing using Reiki and crystals.
9. Get the students to give themselves a Reiki and crystal self-treatment.

I have found there needs to be a time lapse between giving each other a treatment and a self-treatment during a Reiki and Crystal Class. Reiki and Crystal treatments work best when you receive just one treatment per day. However, you can get around this by using a different set of crystals for each treatment i.e., use a quartz set for the treatment and a chalcedony set for the self-treatment or vice versa. The self-treatment (which will be their second Reiki and Crystal treatment for the day) may not be as powerful as the first treatment.

NOTES ON TEACHING 3A (ADVANCED) DEGREE REIKI

Why Teach 3A Reiki

The four Reiki symbols and the three levels of Reiki could be called a complete system that takes someone through the whole process of healing the physical, mental/emotional and spiritual. The 1st Degree of Reiki is primarily the physical level. The 2nd Degree is the mental/emotional level and the 3rd Degree's focus is spiritual. Someone who has done 2nd Degree Reiki for a while often feels incomplete or has an urge to go further. Many people have chosen to discover their spirituality in this lifetime and so they feel compelled to do the 3rd level of Reiki. Often they resist because of the price of Reiki Master training or because they do not want to teach Reiki. 3A can be a good compromise. It has a lower price than Reiki Master training yet attunes the student to the 4th symbol and the 3rd level of Reiki and gives them the opportunity to give temporary Reiki Attunements.

I expect a Reiki Practitioner, who wants to do their Reiki Master/teacher training with me, to have done a 3A class. I have found that the 3A level is a good platform from which to decide whether or not to move on to teaching Reiki. At this level the practitioner discovers whether they enjoy giving Reiki attunements, talking about Reiki to others and using the Usui Reiki Master Symbol. It also helps the student to understand the process of an attunement and to have experience giving attunements so the formulas for the other attunements they have to learn at Master level are easier to learn and understand.

Who to Teach

There is some disagreement between Reiki Masters about who can do 3A Degree of Reiki. One opinion is that anyone who has done 2nd Degree Reiki can do 3A. They make no judgment about whether the student is good enough or ready enough to do the class. The other opinion is that 3A Degree is a very serious step and only certain people can do it. These Reiki Masters hold an interview with the student to determine whether the student is ready to do 3A and sometimes they have a questionnaire for the student to fill out. Others will only teach students the 3A level if they also make a commitment to go on to Reiki Master training.

How you choose your students is entirely up to you. If a Reiki Master went through an interview when they applied for their 3A class it is likely they will set up a similar process for their students.

My preference is not to make a judgment—that the practitioner is better able to judge whether they are ready to move on to this level of Reiki than me. As Reiki Masters, I believe it is our job to teach practitioners, not make their decisions for them. I simply determine whether the person wanting to do 3A knows their 2nd Degree symbols. I do not teach or revise the 2nd Degree symbols in my 3A class. Some Reiki Masters spend an evening prior to the 3A class going over the 2nd Degree Reiki symbols to ensure everyone knows them, or has the same version of symbols as themselves.

How Many Students in a Class

During a 3A Reiki class students are usually taught how to draw and use the Reiki Master Symbol and how to do a Temporary Attunement. Based on my experience I recommend having no more than 4 people in a 3A class. The hard work comes from always being aware of what each person in your class is doing and what point they are at when they are practicing the attunement. People learn at different speeds and also practice at different speeds. You cannot just take notice of the slowest or the fastest in the class. You have to accept that your students will each learn at a different pace and you have to be able to give each one your attention and be aware when someone needs help or is making mistakes. This gets harder to do with each extra person in a class. I find it is hard to watch the Reiki Symbols being drawn by someone else. I have also noticed that when someone asks if they can watch you doing an attunement they invariably close their eyes during the process. It appears to me that the symbols take you into another consciousness where it is very hard for you to keep your eyes open. It takes a lot of effort to stay in this reality while watching the Reiki symbols, which operate in another reality, being drawn.

3rd Degree Reiki—Master & Teacher

If you teach Advanced Reiki, without the Temporary Heart Attunement technique, then it will not matter how many people you have in a class. Advanced Reiki classes often include other techniques such as a crystal grid for absent healing and Qi Gong techniques for directing the energy around your body. The teacher doesn't need to be so focused on each individual student for these subjects as they do when teaching an attunement.

What to Teach in 3A Reiki

As stated above, I do not teach or revise the 2nd Degree symbols in my class. I accept anyone who has done 2nd Degree into my 3A Reiki classes and honor their previous choice of Reiki Master by letting them use the symbols they are attuned to. I do not expect them to change their symbols to the way I do mine.

Because of my lineage, which comes from William Lee Rand via Barbara Pillsbury, I used to teach the Hui Yin point and Violet Breath. It didn't take too long for me to discover I didn't need to use either of these methods and that they had been added into Reiki at a later date, after Mrs. Takata died. I stopped using them and found it didn't make any difference to my attunements. I was glad I no longer have to waddle like a duck while doing attunements.

I teach:
a. The Usui Reiki Master symbol (the Japanese version because of clarity)—how to draw and use it.
b. The breath—when and how to blow during an attunement.
c. Explanation of the attunement—why and where you place your hands.
d. How to do a Temporary Heart Attunement—and give students time to practice.
e. When to use the Temporary Heart Attunement.

I give students plenty of time to practice using the Reiki Master symbol and doing Temporary Heart Attunements.

How to Teach the Reiki Master Symbol

Some students come into the 3A Reiki class expecting the Reiki Master symbol to be very difficult to learn. Their anxiety is usually based on how difficult they found the Distance Symbol during their 2nd Degree class.

When Reiki students first see the Reiki Master symbol they often express relief because it is shorter and less complicated than the Distance Symbol. I usually take the opportunity at this moment to say, *"If you know how to do the Distance Symbol then the Reiki Master Symbol is easy to learn."* This usually eases any resistance a student may have had to learning the Reiki Master Symbol.

There are two strands of belief about the Reiki Master symbol taught at 3A. One is to teach exactly the same symbol as the one used at Reiki Master level and the other is to teach a slightly different Reiki Master symbol. My choice is to teach exactly the same symbol at both 3A and Reiki Master level—this ensures there is no confusion about the Reiki Master symbol. The different Reiki Master symbols have come about because people did not know Japanese and the symbol changed as it was passed down the Reiki lineages. I teach the Japanese version of the Reiki Master symbol. You do not need to be re-attuned to the Japanese version. All you need to do is practice drawing it the Japanese way. You have already been attuned to the symbol when you became a Reiki Master—even if your symbol looks different—it is just a variation of the Japanese symbol, not a different symbol. The Japanese Reiki Master symbol is easy to teach because each part of it is easy to explain.

Drawing the Reiki Master Symbol

Take the student through the first three strokes that mean *Dai* (same as *Tai* in Chinese). The Reiki Master symbol begins much like the Distance symbol and for people who draw the Distance symbol with very little effort or thought, they may find they automatically continue drawing the Distance symbol. To avoid this suggest to your students that they try to make the first downward stroke of the Dai a large curve instead of a straight line. The curve will act as a prompt for the student to continue drawing the strokes of the Reiki Master symbol:

1. First stroke is horizontal—it means one.
2. Second stroke starts above the horizontal line and sweeps down to the left—the line of the body from head to foot.
3. Third stroke starts at the bottom side of the horizontal line and sweeps down to the right—the other leg. Together the 2nd and 3rd strokes of this symbol represent the human body.

3rd Degree Reiki— Master & Teacher

Stand with your feet apart and your hands held out horizontally and show the student that this is where the symbol came from. A person standing so they are balanced. The number one man is usually the chief or king in a society. Hence this symbol came to mean Great. In the East a "Great" person stays in balance no matter what happens to him/her.

The next six strokes are for the Japanese word **Ko**, which means Light.
4. Draw the full length central stroke first.
5. Draw the small half circle on the left.
6. Draw the small diagonal stroke on the right.

These three strokes mean Fire. At the mental/emotional level fire is the passion that you carry within about life, living, yourself, your talents and interests.
7. Draw the horizontal stroke—this stroke can mean 'one' but in this instance it also means 'being carried'—when you carry something it becomes part of you or 'one' with you.
8. Draw the curved stroke on the left (it is like the left curved strokes in the Distance Symbol); this represents a leg standing on the ground.
9. Draw the curved stroke on the right—this stroke is like an L its downward stroke is curved but at the bottom it lengthens out like the bottom of an L; this represents a leg bending at the knee as a person takes a step.

The 5th and 6th steps represent a man walking. The character of Ko comes from a time when light was a burning stick carried by a person. Ko can also mean Torch or Lamp being carried. Today, Ko is used to mean the modern lights that have replaced burning sticks, torches and lamps. This part of the Usui Reiki Master symbol means being able to stay in balance while we are carrying the light; try carrying a tray with a burning candle on it and see how carefully you need to stay balanced.

The third part of the Reiki Master symbol is made up of two symbols— the first symbol represents the sun and the second symbol represents the moon. Together they form the Japanese word **Myo**, which is the same as **Ming** in Chinese. (If you look up the word **Ming** in a Tao dictionary you will find it is considered a very spiritual and special symbol).

The two characters form two boxes. The first character, the sun, is also found in the Distance Symbol. You draw it the same way.

10. Drawing from top to bottom, draw a straight downward stroke.
11. Next draw the top and right side of the box as one stroke. This is because Chinese and Japanese draw with brushes and lifting a brush at the end of the top stoke and then putting the brush back to draw the right side of the box would cause a mess so any strokes that look like a 7 are drawn as one stroke.
12. Draw the horizontal line in the middle. The line can either touch or not touch both sides of the box. It doesn't seem to be important which way you draw it.
13. Draw the stroke that closes off the box at the bottom. The second character of Myo is the moon. You draw it in the same sequence as the symbol for the sun but with longer downward strokes.
14. Drawing from top to bottom, draw a long curved downward stroke.
15. Next draw the top and right side of the box as one stroke. The downward part of this stroke should go down to the same level as the first stroke. You can end the stroke with a tiny upward tick that goes towards the center of the box. This is a brush technique and is not an actual stroke nor does it have any meaning. It is just a nice way to end the stroke.
16. Draw the stroke in the middle—once again it can be drawn so that it either touches or doesn't touch both sides of the box. Draw it at the same level as the same stroke in the sun symbol.
17. Draw the stroke that closes off the box. Draw it at the same level as the stroke in the sun symbol. The two vertical strokes will be longer than the box and make the symbol look like a box on stilts.

Get the student to draw the Reiki Master symbol at least 15 times. If they use colored pens, get them to change colors as this will help with learning the symbol in different areas of the brain. Be patient and give the student plenty of time to practice. Also get them to practice drawing the symbol in the air and with their mind's eye.

Using the Reiki Master Symbol

Treatments

Show the student how to draw the symbol over their body then press it in. They will probably have been taught this at 2nd Degree but go over it again—demonstrating it lets the idea of using the Reiki Master symbol on the body get through to the student. The Reiki Master symbol can be:

1. Drawn at each hand position.
2. Included in a treatment when you are intuitively directed to use it.
3. Drawn as a large symbol over the whole body at the beginning, during and end of a treatment.

Affirmations

All the Reiki symbols can be used to empower affirmations or you can just use the Usui Reiki Master symbol followed by the Power symbol. Ask the student to write their favorite affirmation on a piece of paper and draw all four Reiki symbols on the paper around the affirmation. Get them to hold the paper in their hands and repeat the affirmation to themselves three times, then say the name of the Reiki Master symbol three times.

The name of the Reiki Master symbol has power and can be used without the symbol. This is because the characters within the symbol and the names of the symbol mean the same.

The word Reiki also has a lot of power and energy in it. The word 'Reiki' can be repeated three times at the start and end of an affirmation.

Using the Reiki Master Symbol with other Reiki symbols

Take your students through the various ways you use the Reiki Master symbol. Get them to place all the symbols into the body of another student.

I personally feel that the Reiki Master symbol helps repair damage to the body quickly i.e., torn or injured skin or broken bones, surgery, etc.

Some Reiki Masters ask permission to use this symbol. I don't think this is necessary. I believe that someone asking for a treatment expects the best I can give them and if I feel I should use the Reiki Master symbol then I use it. I have done treatments where the Reiki Master symbol was the only one I used and other treatments where it never crossed my mind to use it.

Healing Crisis

I believe it is important not to give your students ideas about what kind of healing crisis can happen at 3rd Degree. Saying that 'the manure will hit the fan' or 'your marriage will break up' can make a big impression at a vulnerable time. It can emphasize something that may not really be very bad or is hardly there at all. A Reiki class is a time when students are very open to suggestions by the Master. They often take in everything a Master says wholeheartedly without discrimination or judgment. A Master needs to be aware of this and choose their words carefully.

I personally found that the pace of life often increases after a 3A attunement. This increase in pace is simply the clearing up and cleaning out of unfinished business—things that have been allowed to drift or have not been finished or things intended to be done at some stage but never got around to. The attunement gives the energy and impetus to complete these things.

I think it is important to recommend that your students do 21 days of self-treatments during which time they use the Usui Reiki Master symbol at each hand position. This will help them to flow through this change and pace of the energy.

Reiki Guides

It took me a while to get used to the idea that I would be working with guides when I did Reiki attunements. Consequently I believe that you need to take time to discuss this aspect of Reiki with your 3A students.

Ask your students to think about the Higher Beings they want to work with. Reiki Practitioners have worked with the spirit and energy of Jesus Christ, all the various Angels and Archangels, Ascended Reiki Masters, and Spiritual Guides. This part of the class can sometimes generate quite a lot of discussion and may also bring forth names that you have not heard of before. If the student is happy with whom they have chosen for their guides then so be it.

Make your students aware that they can ask their Reiki guides to help them whenever they get stuck during an attunement and that the person receiving the attunement will not mind if their attunement takes a little longer and will probably not notice that you have paused for a moment or two to mentally commune with your guides for instructions.

The Dry Bathing Technique

This technique is really great for disconnecting after a treatment or attunement. I cannot recommend it enough. This technique has only recently been introduced to the West and there are still many students who have not learned how to do it. Although I teach this technique in 1st Degree Reiki classes I also go over it again during all my other Reiki classes. The more it is used the faster and stronger the disconnection. It can be used to disconnect after doing other modalities.

The Temporary Heart Attunement

This attunement is traditionally the first one of the four attunements received at 1st Degree Reiki. Today there are several lineages of Reiki who give one or two attunements at 1st Degree and the attunements used are not the ones that were used for the original four 1st Degree attunements. Over the years, and with different lineages, attunements have changed. The attunement that I teach will probably be different from the attunement you teach. Use the Temporary Heart Attunement that you were taught in your 3A class or during your Reiki Master training. If you have not done 3A Reiki or do not know how to do a Temporary Heart Attunement, make arrangements to sit in on a 3A Reiki class. Alternatively, ask a Reiki Master who knows about Temporary Heart Attunements to teach it to you; don't forget to offer an exchange for the lesson(s).

Make your students aware that the attunement is simply a formula that with practice becomes very easy to do. You need to stress the importance of practice. The Reiki energy may flow like magic from their hands and they don't have to think about it or do much for it to flow but an attunement requires practice. They need to commit the formula for the attunement to memory and that means doing the attunement over and over again until they can do it automatically.

Another point that is important about the attunement is that it is a sacred occasion. It is a time of working with the energies of God or the Sacred. Many people receiving a Reiki attunement, regardless of what degree or whether it is a permanent or temporary attunement, experience it as a profound and spiritual moment in their lives.

Recommend to your students that they treat all Reiki attunements, even temporary ones, as a very special occasion. With that attitude they will also experience it as a profound moment that will extend their own spiritual growth.

Another point that should be stressed is that if an attunement is started it should ALWAYS be finished. A Reiki Practitioner should not stop to do something else during an attunement i.e., to have a drink of water or to answer a phone or door.

Effectiveness of the Heart Attunement

The Heart Attunement is only temporary. How long it is effective depends on the person receiving the attunement. It can last from approximately one week to up to three months. On rare occasions it has been known to last longer. Some Reiki Masters do not like the 3A level of Reiki because they are afraid that a Temporary Attunement may not be temporary. I have never known an occasion when it hasn't been. I have heard of and met some people who claimed their Temporary Heart Attunement was still effective after 3 months. When asked to give proof that they could still channel Reiki they always decline. If the Temporary Heart Attunement is taught correctly it will always be temporary.

Tell your students it is better to underestimate how long a Temporary Heart Attunement will last. They should emphasize to the person about to receive an attunement that it is only temporary and it could be effective from a week to a month.

Teaching The Temporary Heart Attunement

I found the easiest way to teach the Temporary Heart Attunement is to divide it into parts and teach it to the student part by part. As the attunement is a formula it is easy to divide it into parts. Prior to teaching the attunement I spend some time showing students how to draw a Power Symbol in their mouth and then blow it out over the chakras. This part of the class can be lots of fun as students literally get their tongues around it. Here is how I divide up the attunement:

Part 1   Preparing the person receiving the attunement—i.e., how to sit, etc.

Part 2   Setting the intent and preparing yourself to give an attunement.

Part 3	The first part of the attunement i.e., my attunement starts at the back of the receiver.
Part 4	The second part of the attunement i.e., next step of my attunement is at the front of the receiver and blowing on the chakras.
Part 5	The third part of the attunement i.e., third step of my attunement is at the back with hands on the shoulders.
Part 6	The final part of the attunement, i.e., blessing the receiver and ending the attunement.

Take a look at the attunement that you do and break it down into parts. Look for the natural breaks such as moving from one place to another i.e., from the back to the front of the receiver. To teach the attunement:

Show	Stand in front of the class and actually do the part of the attunement you are about to get them to do on a doll or pillow.
Explain	Talk your way through what you are showing them. Explain what you are doing. Repeat showing and explaining at least three times.
Guide	Get the student to do the part you have just demonstrated while you read aloud each movement step by step.
Practice	Get the student to practice the part you have shown them several times. Read the movements aloud for the first two or three practices then get them to do that part while you stay silent.

Once the student(s) have practiced the part you have shown them so they can do it without you telling them what to do, move on to the next part. The repetition can get boring for some students—especially those who have just come along for the certificate and hadn't expected to do too much work. You have to be strict about them doing this practice. You also need to be very attentive during this period and watch what each student is doing. With careful observation you will pick up bad habits and mistakes and will be able to correct them before they become entrenched in that student's practice.

When you are satisfied that the students are reasonably confident about the different parts of the attunement, get them to do a complete attunement. After that give them a break. When the break is over instruct them to do another attunement.

If everything goes well, get them to give each other a temporary heart attunement or, if you only have one student, get them to give you one.

What to Practice Attunements On

The student(s) will need to have something to practice the attunements on. You can ask them to bring along a teddy bear. I have found that there is nearly always a student who forgets to bring something along. For a long time I made calico dolls that the student could use in the class and then take away to practice on. However, this can be very time consuming. I eventually found it too much to stay up until after midnight sewing dolls and making their clothing prior to a class.

The other option, which I now use, is a pillow. I draw hands (left and right on two sheets of paper) and staple the sheets of paper to the pillowcase. The pillow is set on a chair and acts as a receiver during the initial practice of the attunement. When the students get proficient they can then practice on each other.

Other Ways of Doing the Attunement

Self-Attunement

A self-attunement can be used to boost energy, for healing, or to implant a powerful affirmation or intent or because it is a lovely experience. Explain to your students some of the ways of doing a self-attunement. Demonstrate one way of doing a self-attunement. I usually show the students how to do one on their legs.

Distant/Absent Temporary Heart Attunement

You will need to have a discussion in your class about getting permission to send Distant/Absent Attunements. This discussion will probably be quite lively and may push some people's buttons. You will find that the discussion will include how they feel about getting permission for sending Distant/Absent Healing. Although I don't always get permission for Distant/Absent Healing I always get permission to send an attunement. A Distant/Absent Attunement seems to be more effective when the person receiving firstly gives permission and secondly sits in a quiet, meditative state during the time they are told the attunement will take place.

Attunement for 3A/Advanced Reiki

To bring a student into alignment with the 3A/Advanced Reiki level there is one attunement, which is similar to the Reiki Master attunement. It also attunes the student to the Usui Reiki Master symbol. At the beginning of the attunement, when you are preparing yourself for the attunement and setting the intention of the attunement, state the name of the degree and that the student is to be attuned to this level. It is the spiritual guides who determine the level a person is attuned to and what is required for that level. You simply have to continue with the attunement formula you were taught to do for this level of Reiki.

NOTES ON TEACHING REIKI MASTERS/TEACHERS

Who you teach to Reiki Master/Teacher level is your choice. How you teach Reiki Masters and Teachers is also your choice but you will be influenced strongly by how you were taught. Always remember that you have probably taught a lot of people Reiki Master level without knowing it just by the example you set as a Reiki Master. Students in your 1st and 2nd Degree classes will already have made judgments about how they are going to be Reiki Masters based on your behavior as a Reiki Master. When students come to you for Reiki Master/Teacher training they will already have a vision in their minds of how they see themselves as Reiki Masters.

Reiki Masters often wait until they are asked before training someone as a Reiki Master. Some Reiki Masters advertise their Reiki Master classes in newspapers and magazines. Choose the way that suits you best. I recommend you teach just one person Reiki Master first so that you can see how you cope and whether you need to adjust your class or improve it.

I have, from time to time, been warned about the karma of teaching Reiki Masters. This apparently is a fear-based approach designed to put people off teaching too many Reiki Masters. The only karma that I have noticed with teaching Reiki Masters comes about when a Reiki Master does not complete the training of a Master student. This can cause all kinds of problems, mostly built on resentment and anger.

When you take on the training of a Master student I believe you create a contract even if it is only a verbal contract. However, because we are dealing with Reiki, the contract has a spiritual element. You have not just made an agreement between yourself and the student, but also with Reiki to take a person to Reiki Master level. If your verbal contract gets broken, the spiritual one does not. The breaking of a contract needs to have the agreement of all parties; yourself, the student and Reiki. The best way to resolve the dissolving of a Reiki contract is to hold a small ceremony with yourself and the student concerned in which you both declare that the contract is dissolved and to ask Reiki to recognize and accept that the student no longer wants to continue their Reiki training with you. You can include pouring water over each other's hands to wash away the contract or to write it on paper and burn it. If you do not or did not end the arrangement amicably then take some time to do so by sending Absent Healing to provide closure and healing. Use the Distance Symbol to build a connection between yourself, the student and Reiki. Ask that all parties be released from the contract to take your student to Reiki Master level. Use the Reiki Master symbol to ensure there is no negative karma attached to the premature ending of the contract and to bless all concerned.

When to Take on Reiki Master Students

When I was doing my Reiki Master training it was recommended that I wait a year before training someone else to be a Reiki Master. This allows time for you to gain experience in teaching 1st and 2nd Degree Reiki. You can then pass on your own personal experience of teaching Reiki to your Reiki Master students as well as the information you received from your Master lineage. They will also have a lot more respect for what you are teaching if you are firmly grounded in experience.

Being asked by several people if you can teach them to be a Master can be an indication that you are ready to teach that level of Reiki. If you are not sure about it then talk it over with the Reiki Master who taught you or other Reiki Masters. Meditate on why you don't feel ready to teach Master level and then do something about the answer. You may need to re-read notes, sit another course, or just do some basic preparation for the class first to find you are ready to teach a Master student.

Class Content

There really isn't any standardized training for Reiki Master within the overall Reiki community. Each Reiki Master develops their own training for their Master students. This can mean that the length of time for training can range from a few days to a year. Classes can include written assignments, sitting in on a certain number of 1st and 2nd Degree Reiki classes, arranging classes, learning attunements, and sometimes doing other classes such as hypnotherapy, NLP, accelerated learning, counseling and teaching adults. The best way to look at what to use when teaching Reiki Masters is to look at what you liked about your Reiki Master training and what else you would have liked included.

Independence

When you have completed training a Reiki Master and have given them their final Master Attunement then it is time to let the student go and let them stand on their own two feet. Your role is to teach them how to function well as a Reiki Master. It is up to them to learn how to master themselves and their lives. You can show them the tools that you have used in your life—those tools can be Reiki, crystals, psychology, common sense, books you have read and so on. It is their choice whether they use the tools you have shown them. You are not responsible for your Reiki Master students after you have completed their training. They are responsible for their actions and their lives—only in that way can they truly become Masters. You should always encourage them to be independent of you otherwise they will never have the opportunity to truly take on the mantle of Reiki Master. Always release and let go of your Reiki Master students with love and your blessings. Some of your students will leave and you will never see them again and others will remain friends. Always ensure that you treat the Reiki Masters you have trained as equal to you (this can be hard sometimes) and allow them room to hold their own opinions about Reiki and life.

Attunement to Reiki Master

I believe that there may once have been at least six attunements to the 3rd level—one for each of the Buddhas/Kings who sit on the 3rd level of the Healing Buddha mandala. I give my Reiki Master students six attunements to the 3rd level of Reiki. Each of these attunements is to align them to the 3rd Level Buddhas of the Healing Buddha mandala and prepare them for becoming a Reiki Master. On our final day together as Master and Student I give them a Reiki Master attunement which is the same attunement but with the intent that they are attuned to the Reiki Master level of Reiki. Each attunement feels different, with the Reiki Master attunement being very special.

Many Reiki Masters make their Reiki Master attunements very special occasions, which is always appreciated by their students. I ask my students what they would like to happen for their attunement and I try to accommodate them.

I once had a Reiki Master student who wanted to be attuned at the top of a remote hill out in the bush. It would have meant a trek of about an hour, most of it uphill. I wasn't sure if I would be fit enough, however, I agreed then privately asked Reiki to ensure that everything would happen for the highest good of all and to ensure I could cope with whatever happened. The next day it poured with rain so we held the attunement indoors, in a beautiful meditation room, under a stain glass dome, witnessed by a large golden statue of a Buddha. It was perfect.

CONCLUSION

The level of Master in the Western form of Reiki is not an end but a new beginning. To get the most out of this level of Reiki requires work. Not just through teaching others but also by teaching yourself to be a better person. Each student who comes your way will reflect how far you have progressed and what else you need to learn. There will be times when you will do a lot of teaching and other times when you will do little. The quiet times are there for you to work on yourself—giving you time to do more self-treatments, absent healing, to attend support groups, to read books and develop relationships. When you are ready to move on to another level of Mastership students will find you again.

If you have chosen not to teach Reiki classes you will find that you will be given opportunities to be an example of how Reiki works in someone's life, or you may be invited to give talks about Reiki to others, or to act as a leader of a Reiki group. Once you have accepted the title of Reiki Master there is no going back. You can choose to stagnate, to not do any further learning or to not use Reiki anymore. This can mean you will be jolted out of this attitude at some time by something that forces you to use Reiki again.

Reiki is not just for those who are sick or unhappy. It is also a tool for lifting you up to higher levels of yourself and to ensure that you travel the pathway of this lifetime of yours in the best way you can. As you learn to enjoy life, be grateful for life and to see all of life as one, the world will become a magical place that blesses you with love and abundance.

RECOMMENDED READING

Re-read all of the Reiki books that you have collected while learning Reiki. Go to your public library and read the Reiki books they have that you do not have. You may not need all the information contained in the books but it will provide you with a good basic background on Reiki that will help support you in your role as a Reiki Master and Reiki Teacher.

Continue to read books and attend classes about relationships, human nature, energy work, health and anything that you find interesting and relevant to you. It is said you should travel from joy to joy and do what interests and excites you. You never know where it will take you but it will always be interesting and fun.

May your journey joyfully continue

In the light and love of Reiki . . .

Index